100 Slow Cooker Recipes for you: Cookbook how to cook healthy meals for Weight Loss

Helena Smith

Have you ever wanted to lose weight while still enjoying those tasty meals without having to go through all those exhausting diets? It may seem farfetched, but nevertheless it is possible to lose weight without starving yourself. There is no need to exhaust your body with useless diets. It is possible to get rid of excessive weight just by changing your eating habits!

This is the first book from the series «Lose weight easy, tasty and without starving», that will help its readers to take the first step in achieving their goal of a healthier body.

Contents

The Slow Cooker: What You Need to Know 7
Breakfast 10
    Nutmeg-Infused Pumpkin Bread 10
    Apple Granola Crumble 11
    Pecan Granola 12
    Cinnamon Granola 14
    Carrot Cake and Zucchini Break Oatmeal 15
    Apple Pie Oatmeal 16
    Fruit, Nuts and Spice Oatmeal 17
    Breakfast Casserole #1 18
    Breakfast Casserole #2 19
    Blueberry and Chia Quinoa 20
    Steel-cut Oats with Blueberries and Bananas 21
    Huevos Rancheros 22
    Spinach and Mozzarella Frittata 23
    Veggie Omelette 24
    Coconut Rice Pudding with Mangoes and Pistachio Nuts 26
    Lemon Cornmeal Poppy Seed Bread 27
    Vanilla Bean and Almond French Toast 28
    Tater Tot Egg Bake 29
    Breakfast Grit 30
    Stuffed Bell Peppers 31
    Quinoa Energy Bar 32
    Banana Bread 33
    Coconut Brown Rice Pudding 35
    Loaded Potato Soap 36
Dinner 38
    Lemony Pork Roast 38
    BBQ Pulled Pork 39
    Chilli Beans and Sweet Potato 40

Chicken Stock 41
Vegetable Pizza 42
Chicken and Dumplings 43
Tropical Chicken Dinner 44
Chicken Marrakesh 44
Chicken Tinga 45
Chicken Stroganoff 47
Eggplant Parmesan 47
South-western Vegetarian Dinner 49
Cacciatore Chicken 50
Pepper Steak 51
Vegetarian Chilli 52
Pork and Sauerkraut with Apples 53
Yummy Chuck Roast 54
Cabbage Rolls 55
Beer Braised Chicken 56
Tarragon Lamb Shanks with Cannellini Beans 57
Pesto Lasagne with Spinach and Mushrooms 58
Cassoulet 59
Creamy Tortellini Soup 60
Shio Ramen and Chilli Oil 61
Red Pepper, Feta and Kale Frittata 63
Ropa Vieja 64
Turkey Mole Tacos 65
Chicken and Vegetable Soup 66
French Dip Sandwiches 67
Chicken Tortilla Soup 68
Tex-Mex Casserole 69
Moroccan Chicken and Squash 70
Salmon with Cilantro and Lime 71
Steak Roulade with Provolone 72
Ham with Barbeque Beans 74
Salmon Chowder with Dill 75

Corned Beef and Cabbage 76
Paprika Goulash 77
Garlic Butter Tilapia 78
Posole 79
Barley and Chickpea Risotto 80
Supper 81
Rabbit Stew 82
Cheesy Mashed Potatoes 83
Onion Dip in French Style 84
Baked Beans 85
Creamed Corn 86
Corn Chowder 87
Split Pea Soup 87
Peach Cobbler 89
Tapioca Pudding 90
Green Bean Risotto 91
White Bean Stew 92
Cawl Cennin (Leek Soup) 94
French Onion Soup 95
Seafood Cioppino 96
Broccoli and Cheese Soup 97
Lentil Stew with Butternut Squash 98
Butternut Squash Stew 99
Red Lentil Curry 100
Vindaloo Vegetables 102
Mexican Quinoa 103
Lemon Rosemary Lentil Soup 105
Black Bean Soup 106
Butter Chickpeas and Tofu 107
Chana Masala 108
Chicken Chilli 109
Chicken Fajitas 110
Super food Soup 111

Pinto & Black Bean Chilli 111
Quinoa Risotto 112
Chicken Soup 113
Spinach and Artichoke Chicken 114
Fiesta Chicken Soup 115
Curly Coley 116
Butternut Squash and Parsnip Soup 116
Lemon Rosemary Beets 117

The Slow Cooker: What You Need to Know

Slow Cookers are cheap, efficient to use, and very effective when it comes to making good use of budget ingredients. With slow cookers, you make fewer efforts and get the healthiest foods. What more could you ask for?

The technique used to cook food in a slow cooker includes preparation of the meal in hot liquid, usually for long hours, until the bubble formation in the food is stopped. Slow cooker requires a lot less water than conventional cookers as the liquid which evaporates, stays inside, hence, having the cooker filled up half or two-thirds of the maximum are good enough.

Since the ingredients (vegetables, meat, seasoning) are cooked for long hours in either low or medium heat settings, it brings out the natural taste and flavor in the food, retaining the natural juices and preserving the nutrition which as a result bestows with a healthy mind and body.

Generally, there are a few guidelines that you need to follow while using a slow cooker. These are:

Safety First
Slow cooker doesn't require the cook to be around while the meal is prepared and as a result, it is a great choice for working females who would not want to spend time in preparation of food after spending long hours at work and taking care of a lot of other family and personal activities. It is advised to wear oven mitts as the cooker as well as lid tends to get very hot after long hours cooking. Slow cookers shouldn't be more than half or two-third full as it can be dangerous. Avoid putting cooker inserts on gas stoves, electrical burner or freezer. Do not remove the lid while preparing the food until the required time for preparation is over. Position it near an outlet & tries to keep it approximately 6" (15.2 cms) away from the materials, walls or any other kitchen appliances.

Prepare The Recipe

Food is prepared at a comparatively low temperature; however, the preparation takes a couple of hours than usual, when compared to boiling, frying or baking the food. It is advised to cover the device with glass lid while preparing food. It is manufactured in different varieties and capacities ranging from a 500 ML to as far as 7 Liters.

It gives users an option for different heat settings such as low, medium, high and in a few devices a setting popularly known as 'keep warm'.

Adding oil or having fat on the meat isn't required in a slow cooker else you'll find oil in the stew/dish. It is advised to trim the fat prior to the cooking. This would also result in a healthier output.

Put the Ingredients into a Slow Cooker
For optimum results, slow cookers shouldn't be more than half or two-third full as it can be dangerous. You don't need to add plenty of water as very little liquid evaporates during the cooking process. For easy clean up; it's suggested to line the crock of your slow cooker with an aluminium foil.

Put the Lid On
It is advised to cover the pot with the lid because the vapour produced doesn't evaporate hence the vitamins, minerals and other essential nutrients which are water soluble, don't leave the food. The liquid, in the form of vapour also assists with the transfer of heat from the pot walls to the ingredients that gives a natural and distinct flavor to the dish.

For these reasons the lid should be snuggled appropriately to the top of the pot. Basic cookers requires the user to change the heat and temperature modes manually, however, the advanced ones does it automatically.

Set the Cooking Time
Root vegetables usually take longer than the meat and other vegetables to cook, hence, it is advised to keep them at the bottom of the cooker. It gives users an option for different heat settings such as low, medium, high and in a few devices a setting popularly known as 'keep warm'.

If you want to cook your recipe for 8 to 10 hours, then you can always choose the low-heat settings. This setting allows you to cook the food gently, which often results in more tender vegetables and meat. However, if you want your food to be prepared in 4 to 6 hours then feel free to choose the high-heat settings.

The Finished Product

Many modern slow cookers gives an option for different heat settings such as low, medium, high and in a few devices a setting popularly known as 'keep warm'. According to its name, it keeps the meal warm once the preset time is achieved by switching modes on itself. Hence, you wouldn't have to warm, the dish separately before serving.

Also, in most of the devices, once the food is cooked, the device by itself changes the mode to 'keep warm' to ensure the food isn't overcooked and is ready to be served once it is out of the cooker.

Breakfast

Nutmeg-Infused Pumpkin Bread

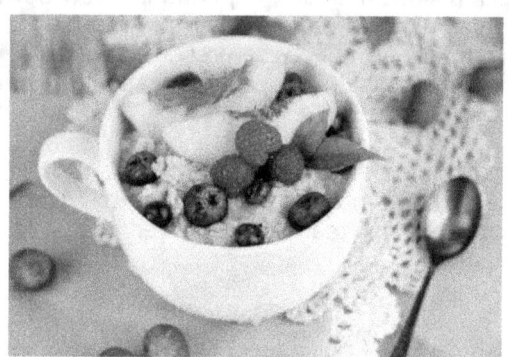

Prep Time: 20 minutes
Cook Time: 165 minutes
Total Time: 185 minutes
Servings: 16
Calories per serving: 220

Suitable for Vegetarians

Ingredients
- ¾ cup white flour, preferably whole-wheat
- 4 egg whites, large
- ¾ cup apple juice concentrate
- 2 oz. toasted pecan pieces, unsalted
- ¼ tsp. ground allspice
- 2 tsp. baking powder
- ½ tsp. baking soda
- 1 cup pumpkin, cooked & puréed
- ½ cup maple sugar flakes
- 1 tsp. ground nutmeg
- ½ cup plain Greek yoghurt, non-fat
- Olive Oil Cooking Spray

Directions
- Coat a non-stick loaf pan lightly with the cooking spray; set aside.
- Over moderate heat settings in a large-sized saucepan; heat the apple concentrate juice until starts boiling; set aside and let sit for a couple of minutes.
- In the meantime; whisk flour together with maple sugar flakes, baking soda, baking powder, allspice, nutmeg &salt in a large-sized bowl.
- Thoroughly combine pumpkin with egg whites, yoghurt, vanilla and safflower oil in a separate bowl until combined well.
- Add the pecans and pumpkin mixture to the flour mixture; give everything a good stir until you can't see the flour anymore; don't over mix the ingredients.
- Spoon it into the bottom of a slow cooker & using a spatula or spoon; smooth the top.
- Add mixture to the slow cooker. Cover &cook for 2 hours &15 minutes on the high heat setting until a wooden toothpick comes out clean.

When the cooking time completes; let cool for several minutes until you can handle it easily & then cut into 16 pieces.

Apple Granola Crumble

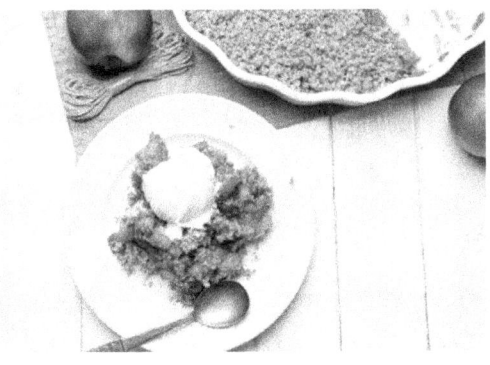

Prep Time: 15 minutes
Cook Time: 240 minutes
Total Time: 255 minutes
Servings: 3 Bowls
Calories per serving: 382

Suitable for Vegetarians

Ingredients
- 2 apples, preferably Granny Smith; peeled, cored & cut into thick slices; then cut into small chunks
- ¼ cup apple juice
- 1 cup granola cereal (½ bran flakes mixed with ½ cup granola cereal)
- ½ tsp. ground nutmeg
- 2 tbsp. butter, dairy-free
- ⅛ cup maple syrup
- 1 tsp. ground cinnamon

Directions
- Put everything together into the bottom of your slow cooker; give everything a good stir.
- Lock the lid to its place & cook on low-heat settings for 4 hours.

Pecan Granola

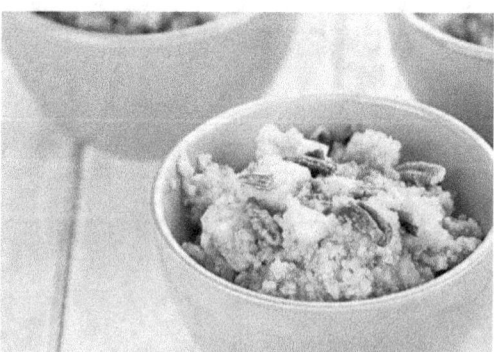

Prep Time: 5 minutes

Cook Time: 180 minutes
Total Time: 185 minutes
Servings: 6
Calories per serving: 417

Suitable for Vegetarians

Ingredients
- 6 tbsp. applesauce
- 1 tsp. ground cinnamon
- ¼ tsp. vanilla extract
- 3 cups rolled oats
- ¼ tsp. maple extract
- 1 cup Medjool dates, pitted & chopped
- ¼ cup pure maple syrup
- 1 cup chopped pecans
- ¼ tsp. salt

Optional Ingredients
- 1 tbsp. Hemp seed hearts
- 2 tbsp. Brown sugar
- 1 tbsp. Chia seeds

Directions
- Pour applesauce together with brown sugar, maple syrup, hemp hearts, vanilla, cinnamon, maple extracts, Chia seeds & salt into the bottom of your slow cooker; give everything a good stir until combined well and then add pecans and oats; stir again to mix.
- Cook for 3 hours on the high setting in slow cooker; keep an eye on everything, don't let it burn. If required, stir occasionally.
- Transfer the cooked granola on a parchment paper lined baking sheet and let cool at room temperature.
- Serve immediately or store in an airtight container.

Cinnamon Granola

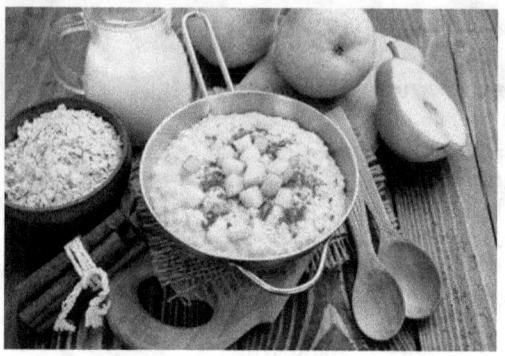

Prep Time: 10 minutes
Cook Time: 180 minutes
Total Time: 190 minutes
Servings: 3-4
Calories per serving: 220

Suitable for Vegetarians

Ingredients
- 3 cups oats, uncooked
- ¼ cup maple syrup
- 6 tbsp. applesauce
- ¼ tsp. almond extract
- 2 tbsp. brown sugar
- 1 tsp. cinnamon
- ¼ tsp. salt

Optional Ingredients
- 1 cup each date and pecans, chopped

Directions

- Put everything together (except oats, dates &pecans) into the bottom of your slow cooker; mix well.
- Place the lid; slightly leaving it ajar so that the steam can escape. Cook for 3 hours on high-heat settings, stirring occasionally.

- Add the oats, dates and pecans during the last 30 minutes of cooking.

Spoon the granola onto a baking sheet lined with the parchment paper and let cool. Cut it into pieces and serve immediately or store them in an airtight container.

Carrot Cake and Zucchini Break Oatmeal

Prep Time: 10 minutes
Cook Time: 420 minutes (approx.)
Total Time: 430 minutes (approx.)
Servings: 2-4
Calories per serving: 118

Suitable for Vegetarians

Ingredients
- ½ cup gluten-free oats, steel-cut
- ½ zucchini, small, peeled & grated
- ⅛ tbsp. nutmeg
- 1½ cups vanilla-flavoured milk, non-dairy
- ¼ cup pecans, chopped
- ⅛ tbsp. ground cloves
- 1 carrot, small, grated
- ½ tsp. cinnamon
- 2 tbsp. maple syrup or brown sugar
- ⅛ tbsp. salt

Optional Ingredients
- 1 tsp. vanilla extract, pure

Directions
- Lightly coat the bottom of your slow cooker with oil.
- Add everything together (except pecans) into the bottom of your slow cooker.
- Cook for 6 to 8 hours on low-heat settings.
- Once done; give everything a good stir & top with the chopped pecans. Serve and enjoy.

Apple Pie Oatmeal

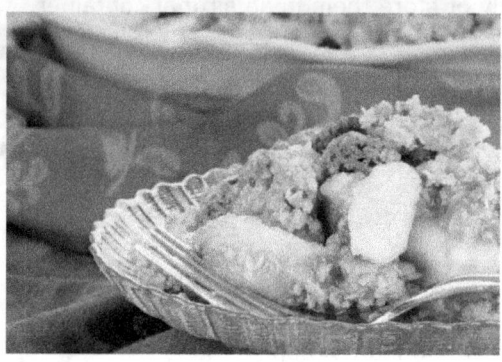

Prep Time: 10 minutes
Cook Time: 240 minutes (approx.)
Total Time: 250 minutes (approx.)
Servings: 12
Calories per serving: 78

Suitable for Vegetarians

Ingredients
- 3 apples, medium, diced
- 1 cup oats, preferably steel-cut
- ½ tsp. ground cinnamon
- 1 cup apple juice
- 3 cups water

Directions
- Pour water into the bottom of your slow-cooker and then add the oats together with diced apples, cinnamon and apple juice; give everything a good stir.
- Cook for 4 to 5 hours on the low-heat settings until the oats are tender & you get your preferred texture, stirring occasionally.

Fruit, Nuts and Spice Oatmeal

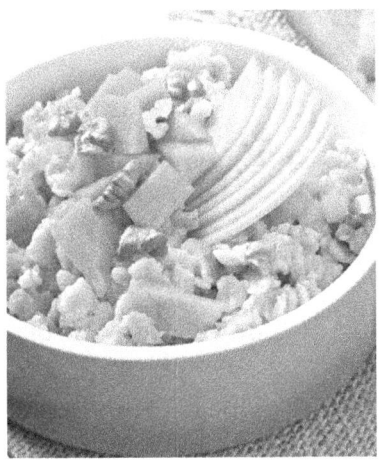

Prep Time: 10 minutes
Cook Time: 480 minutes
Total Time: 490 minutes
Servings: 8
Calories per serving: 326

Suitable for Vegetarians

Ingredients

- 2 cups oats, steel-cut
- 1 tbsp. ground cinnamon
- 2 cups apple, diced
- 1 cup cranberries, dried
- ½ cup pecans, chopped
- 1 cup milk
- ½ cup almonds, slivered
- 2 tsp. butter
- 1 tsp. pumpkin pie spice
- 3 cups water

Directions

- Place oats together with pecans, diced apple, pumpkin pie spice, almonds, cranberries, milk, water, butter and cinnamon in the bottom of your slow cooker; give everything a good stir until evenly mixed.
- Cook for 8 hours or for overnight on the low-heat settings.

Breakfast Casserole #1

Prep Time: 15 minutes
Cooker Time: 420 minutes (approx.)
Total Time: 435 minutes (approx.)
Servings: 10-12
Calories per serving: 382

Ingredients
- 1 cheddar cheese, shredded (16 oz.)
- 12 eggs, large
- 1 bag hash brown potatoes, frozen & thawed (26 oz) or 4 medium-sized potatoes, raw, diced
- 1 pork sausages (16 oz.)
- 2 tbsp. black pepper
- 1 cup milk
- Olive Oil cooking spray
- 1 tsp. salt

Optional Ingredients
- 1 onion, medium
- 2 mushrooms
- 1 green pepper
- 1 tbsp. ground mustard

Directions
- Coat the crock of your slow cooker lightly with the cooking oil.
- Evenly cut the green pepper, mushrooms and onion.
- Spread the diced potatoes (or hash brown potatoes) into the bottom and then spread ½ of shredded cheddar cheese on top of the potatoes.

- Over medium-high heat settings in a large skillet; cook the sausage for 5 to 7 minutes, until browned; cut the cooked sausage into pieces and discard the grease. Spread the sausage on top of hash browns topped with cheddar and then top everything with cheddar cheese again.
- Beat eggs with milk and then add the ground mustard; season the mix lightly with black pepper and salt; mix well. Pour the mixture on top of cheese layer.
- Cook for 6 to 8 hours on the low-heat settings.

Breakfast Casserole #2

Prep Time: 15 minutes
Cook Time: 240 minutes
Total Time: 255 minutes
Servings: 10
Calories per serving: 320

Ingredients
- 4 bacon strips, cooked
- 8 eggs, large
- ¾ cup milk
- 4 egg whites
- ½ tsp. garlic salt
- 6 oz. cheddar cheese
- ½ tsp. pepper
- 1 head of broccoli, small, chopped
- 2 tsp. mustard, stone-ground
- 1 bag hash browns, frozen & thawed (26 oz.) or 4 potatoes, raw
- ½ onion, medium, chopped
- 2 bell peppers, chopped
- 1 tsp. salt

Directions
- Whisk the egg whites together with whole eggs, garlic, mustard, milk, pepper and salt in a medium-sized bowl; whisk well &set aside.

- Grease the bottom of your slow cooker lightly and then place half of the potatoes. Layer with half the bacon, bell peppers, chopped onion, cheese, and broccoli. Add remaining hash browns and then top it with bacon, cheese and the leftover veggies. Pour the egg mixture completely over the top.
- Cover and cook on low-heat settings for 4 hours.

Blueberry and Chia Quinoa

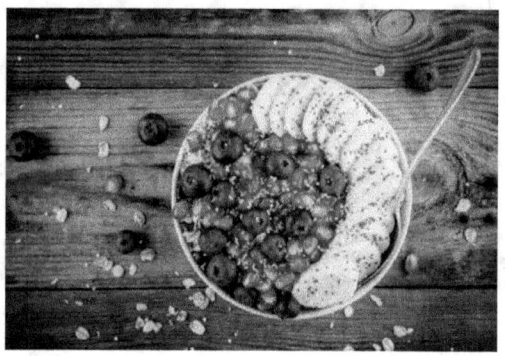

Prep Time: 5 minutes
Cook Time: 390minutes (approx.)
Total Time: 395 minutes (approx.)
Servings: 6
Calories per serving: 381

Suitable for Vegetarians

Ingredients
- 2 cups quinoa
- 4 cups soy milk
- ⅓ cup honey
- 2 cups blueberries, fresh
- 4 cups water
- ⅓ cup Chia seeds

Directions
- Pour the soy milk together with blueberries, quinoa, water, honey and Chia seeds in the bottom of your slow cooker; give everything a good stir until evenly mixed.
- Cook for 6 to 7 hours on low-heat settings. Serve and enjoy.

Steel-cut Oats with Blueberries and Bananas

Prep Time: 10 minutes
Cook time: 420 minutes
Total Time: 430 minutes
Servings: 4
Calories per serving: 315

Suitable for Vegetarians

Ingredients
- 2 tsp. vanilla extract
- 2 cups almond milk
- 1 cup oats, preferably steel-cut
- 2 cups blueberries, fresh
- 2 bananas, ripe, mashed
- 1 tsp. ground cinnamon
- 2 tbsp. honey
- 2 cups water
- ¼ tsp. salt

Directions
- Put everything together into the bottom of your slow cooker (adding the blueberries in the last); give everything a good stir.
- Cook for 6 to 8 hours on the low-heat settings.

Huevos Rancheros

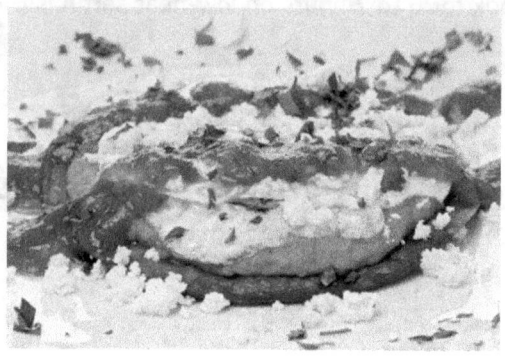

Prep Time: 15 minutes
Cook Time: 120 minutes
Total Time: 135 minutes
Servings: 8
Calories per serving: 500

Suitable for Vegetarians

Ingredients
- 4 oz. green chilli peppers, chopped
- 1 cup half-and-half
- 10 eggs, large
- ½ tsp. anchor-chilli powder
- 12 oz. Monterey jack cheese, shredded
- 1 clove garlic, minced
- 8 corn tortillas
- ½ tsp. black pepper
- 10 oz. taco sauce
- non-stick cooking spray

For Garnish:
- Avocado, scallions, lime and cilantro

Directions
- Lightly coat the inside of your slow cooker with the non-stick cooking spray.

- Beat eggs with 8 ounces cheese, half-and-half, chilli powder and pepper in a large bowl. Stir in the chillies and garlic. Pour the mixture into the slow cooker; cook for 2 hours on the low-heat settings. Make sure that the edges don't burn, feel free to check it occasionally.
- Carefully remove the lid & pour taco sauce completely over the eggs, evenly cover the eggs using the back of a large spoon. Scatter the leftover cheese all over and then place the lid again; continue to cook for 15 minutes more on low heat settings.
- Let it slightly cool and then cut into wedges. Serve on tortillas, preferably warmed. Garnish with sliced avocado and scallions, chopped cilantro & finally a squirt of fresh lime juice.

Spinach and Mozzarella Frittata

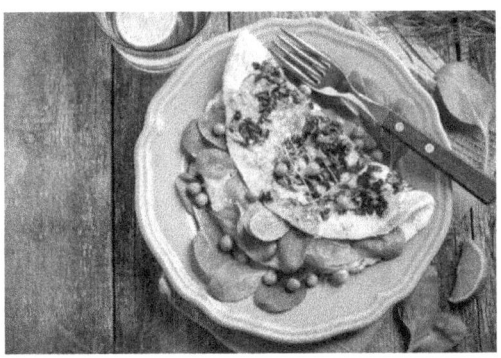

Prep Time: 5 minutes
Cook Time: 90 minutes (approx.)
Total Time: 95 minutes (approx.)
Servings: 6
Calories per serving: 139
Suitable for Vegetarians

Ingredients
- 1 cup baby spinach, fresh, chopped, stems removed

- ½ cup onion, diced
- 1 Roma tomato, diced
- 3 eggs, large
- ¼ tsp. white pepper
- 1 cup mozzarella cheese, shredded
- 3 egg whites, large
- ¼ tbsp. black pepper
- 2 tbsp. milk, preferably 1%
- 1 tbsp. extra virgin olive oil
- ¼ tbsp. salt or to taste

Directions
- Over medium heat settings in a small skillet; heat the oil until hot and then sauté the onion for a couple of minutes, until tender.
- Lightly coat the inside of your slow cooker with the non-stick cooking spray or canola oil.
- Combine onion together with ¾ cup mozzarella cheese & the leftover ingredients in a large bowl. Whisk until evenly combined and then pour the mixture completely all into the slow cooker.
- Sprinkle the leftover cheese over the top. Cover & cook until the eggs are set & a wooden toothpick comes out clean, for 1 to 1½ hours on low heat settings.

Veggie Omelette

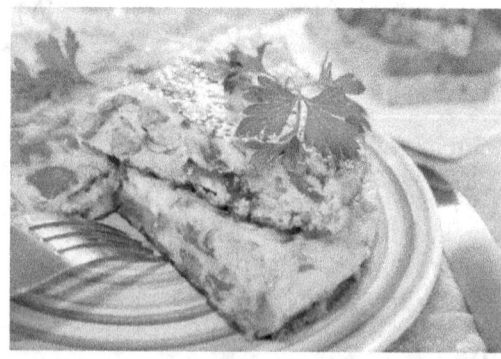

Prep Time: 5 minutes
Cook Time: 120 minutes
Total Time: 125 minutes
Servings: 8
Calories per serving: 280

Suitable for Vegetarians

Ingredients

- 6 eggs, large
- 1 cup broccoli florets
- ⅛ tsp. garlic powder or to taste
- 1 red bell pepper, sliced thinly
- ⅛ tsp. ground pepper or to taste
- 1 small onion, chopped finely
- Olive oil cooking spray
- ½ cup milk
- 1 clove garlic, minced
- ⅛ tsp. chilli powder or to taste
- chopped tomatoes, shredded cheddar cheese, fresh parsley, and chopped onions
- ¼ tsp. salt

Directions

- Lightly coat the inside of your slow cooker with the cooking spray; set aside.
- Combine eggs together with milk, garlic powder, chilli powder, pepper and salt in a large-sized mixing bowl. Beat the mixture using a whisk or egg beaters until well combined and mixed.
- Transfer the egg mixture to the slow cooker and then add sliced peppers, broccoli florets, garlic and onions in the slow cooker; give everything a good stir.
- Cover &cook until the eggs are done and a toothpick comes out clean, for 2 hours on high-heat settings, don't forget to check it often and don't let it burn.
- Sprinkle with cheese; cover & then let stand until the cheese is melted, for a couple of minutes.
- Turn the slow cooker off & cut the omelette into wedges.
- Transfer the wedges to a large-sized serving plate; garnish the plate with chopped onions, chopped tomatoes & fresh parsley. Serve& enjoy.

Coconut Rice Pudding with Mangoes and Pistachio Nuts

Prep Time: 5 minutes
Cook Time: 210 minutes
Total Time: 215 minutes
Servings: 6
Calories per serving: 188

Suitable for Vegetarians

Ingredients
- 1½ cups coconut milk
- 4-8 tsp. pistachio nuts, raw
- ½ cup rice
- 1 cup mango slices
- ½ cup water
- 3 tbsp. honey
- ⅛ tsp. salt

Directions
- Add coconut milk together with rice, water, salt and sugar to your slow cooker. Cover & cook for 3 to 4 hours on low heat settings, stirring every now and then.
- Turn the heat off when you get your desired consistency of pudding and the rice is cooked.
- Serve with some mango slices on top and a sprinkle of raw pistachio nuts.

Lemon Cornmeal Poppy Seed Bread

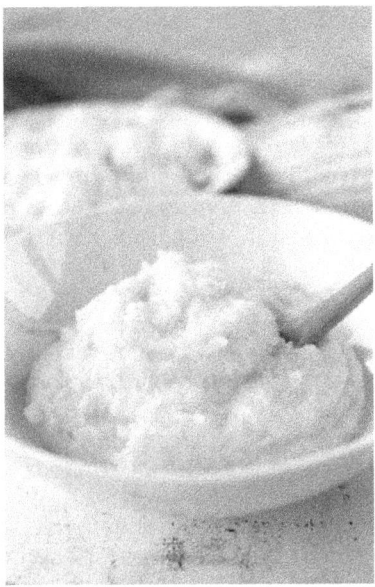

Prep Time: 15 minutes
Cook Time: 190 minutes
Total Time: 205 minutes
Servings: 16
Calories per serving: 220

Suitable for Vegetarians

Ingredients
- Olive oil cooking spray
- 2 tbsp. all-purpose flour
- ½ cup butter, melted
- 3 tsp. baking powder
- ½ cup powdered sugar, for glaze
- 1cup granulated sugar
- 2 tbsp. lemon juice, fresh
- ½ cup yellow cornmeal
- 3eggs, large
- 1 tbsp. lemon peel, finely shredded
- 2 tbsp. poppy seed

- ¾ cup milk
- 2 ½ tsp. lemon juice, fresh, for glaze
- ½ tsp. salt

Directions
- Lightly coat the inside of your slow cooker with the cooking spray.
- Stir flour together with poppy seed, cornmeal, baking powder &salt in a large-sized bowl, until mixed well.
- Mix the leftover ingredients (don't add the fresh lemon juice and powdered sugar) in a separate bowl until combined well. Transfer this mixture into the flour mixture; give everything a good stir until just combined. Spoon the mixture into the slow cooker.
- Cook until a wooden toothpick comes out clean, for 1 hour 40 minutes to 2 hours on high setting settings. Let cool for a couple of minutes.
- Using a thin metal spatula; loosen the edge of the bread. Remove the bread from your slow cooker and transfer it to a cooling rack to cool completely.
- Mix the entire glaze ingredients together in a small bowl, until smooth and gets a consistency of thick syrup. Drizzle the mixture on top of the bread.

Vanilla Bean and Almond French Toast

Prep Time: 10 minutes
Cook Time: 480 minutes
Total Time: 490 minutes
Servings: 8
Calories per serving: 147

Suitable for Vegetarians

Ingredients
- 2 cups whole milk
- 1 vanilla bean, beans only
- 2 cups heavy cream

- 1 tsp. ground cinnamon
- 8 eggs, large
- 1 loaf of challah bread; sliced into ½" slices
- 5 tsp. honey
- 1 tsp. almond extract
- ⅛ tbsp. common salt

Directions
- Grease the inside of your slow-cooker lightly with the cooking spray.
- Arrange the bread slices in the slow-cooker; it's okay if they overlap each other.
- Whisk the remaining ingredients together in a large bowl, until combined well and then pour the mixture into the slow cooker over the Challah bread; pushing the bread down and make sure it's submerged completely.
- Cover and cook on low heat settings for 8 hours.
- Let the French toast to slightly cool and then cut into pieces.

Tater Tot Egg Bake

Prep Time: 15 minutes
Cook Time: 480 minutes
Total Time: 490 minutes
Servings: 6-8
Calories per serving: 217

Ingredients
- 4 tbsp. all-purpose flour
- 1 package tater tots (30 oz.)
- 2 onions, medium, chopped
- ¼ cup parmesan cheese, grated
- 1 cup milk
- 12 eggs, large
- 2 cups cheddar cheese, shredded
- 6 oz. bacon, diced
- ½ tsp. pepper
- 1 tsp. salt

Directions

- Layer 1/3 of the Tots, bacon, cheeses and onions in a greased slow cooker, preferably 5-quart or larger-sized. Repeat these layers two more times; it's important for you to end these layers with the cheese layer.
- Whisk the leftover ingredients together in a large-sized mixing bowl; whisk well and then transfer the mixture on top of the ingredients in the slow cooker.
- Cover & cook for 7 to 8 hours on low heat settings or for overnight.
- Serve and enjoy.

Breakfast Grit

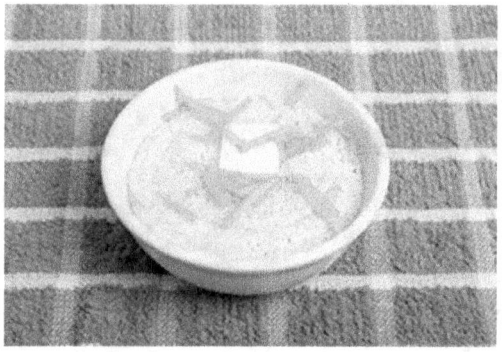

Prep Time: 5 minutes
Cook Time: 480 minutes
Total Time: 480 minutes
Servings: 8
Calories per serving: 150

Suitable for Vegetarians

Ingredients

- 4-6 tbsp. butter, cut into 1 tbsp. sized pieces
- 1½ cup stone ground grits

- olive oil cooking spray
- ½ cup sharp cheddar cheese, shredded
- 6 cups water
- ½ tsp. freshly ground black pepper, to taste
- 2 tsp. salt

Directions
- Lightly coat the inside of a slow cooker, preferably 6-quarts with the cooking spray.
- Add grits together with water and salt in the bottom of your slow cooker; give everything a good stir. Cover &cook for 7 to 8 hours on low heat settings.
- Carefully remove the lid and then scatter butter over the top. Stir the grits using a whisk until the butter melts completely.
- Sprinkle cheese over the top & then sprinkle pepper to taste.

Stuffed Bell Peppers

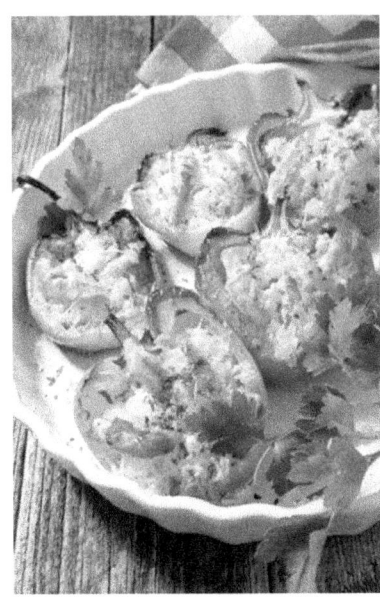

Prep Time: 5 minutes
Cook Time: 240 minutes
Total Time: 245 minutes
Servings: 4
Calories per serving: 209

Ingredients
- 4 bacon slices, uncooked, crumbled
- ½ cup milk
- 4 bell peppers, halved &seeded
- ⅛ cup frozen spinach, thawed & chopped
- 2 tbsp. onion, chopped
- 1 cup cheese
- 5 eggs, large
- ¾ tsp. salt

Directions
- Line your slow cooker with a tin foil and then fill the cooker with the peppers.
- Combine eggs together with spinach, milk, green onion, bacon, cheese & salt in a medium-sized bowl; whisk until well combined. Transfer the mixture into the slow cooker.
- Cook until the eggs are set, for 3 to 4 hours, on low heat settings.

Quinoa Energy Bar

Prep Time: 10 minutes
Cook Time: 240 minutes
Total Time: 250 minutes
Servings: 8
Calories per serving: 170

Suitable for Vegetarians

Ingredients
- 1/3 cup almonds, roasted, chopped roughly
- 2 tbsp. pure maple syrup

- ½ tsp. cinnamon
- 1 cup almond-vanilla milk, unsweetened
- ½ cup raisins
- 2 tbsp. almond butter
- 1/3 cup quinoa, uncooked
- 2 eggs, large
- 1/3 cup apples, dried, chopped roughly
- 2 tbsp. chia seeds
- olive oil cooking spray
- ⅛ tbsp. salt

Directions

- Lightly coat the bottom of your slow cooker, preferably 5-quarts or more with the cooking spray & then fit a parchment paper piece in the bottom of it. Coat the parchment paper with the cooking spray as well; pressing it down and make sure it adheres to it.
- Combine almond butter together with the maple syrup in a large-sized micro-wave safe bowl; heat until the butter is almost creamy, for half a minute.
- Whisk the maple syrup together with the almond butter. Then, whisk in the cinnamon, almond milk & salt; whisk well until the almond butter is completely incorporated with the milk.
- Slowly whisk in the eggs until combined well and then thoroughly stir in the leftover ingredients.
- Transfer the mixture into the prepared slow cooker &cook for 3 ½ to 4 hours, until the top of the bars is just set, on low heat settings.
- Run a sharp knife around the edges of the bars & then remove the bowl from the slow cooker. Let cool at room temperature for a couple of minutes and then place the bowl in a refrigerator until completely cool.
- Cut into bars. Serve & enjoy.

Banana Bread

Prep Time: 30 minutes
Cook Time: 240 minutes
Total Time: 270 minutes

Servings: 4
Calories per serving: 190

Suitable for Vegetarians

Ingredients
- 3 bananas, mashed
- ½ cup butter, softened &cubed
- 2 cups all-purpose flour
- 1 cup nuts
- ½ tsp. baking soda
- 1 tsp. baking powder
- 2 whole eggs, large
- 1 cup granulated sugar
- ½ tsp. salt

Directions
- Mix eggs together with butter and sugar in a large-sized bowl.
- Add 1 cup of flour followed by baking soda, baking powder and salt; mix well and then the remaining flour; mix well until the Mixture appears to be thick.
- Add the mashed bananas into the mixture; mix well.
- Lightly coat the bottom of your slow cooker with the butter.
- Cook on low heat settings until the top turns out to be slightly browned, for 4 hours.
- Remove the bread carefully from slow cooker. Cut into pieces; serve& enjoy.

Coconut Brown Rice Pudding

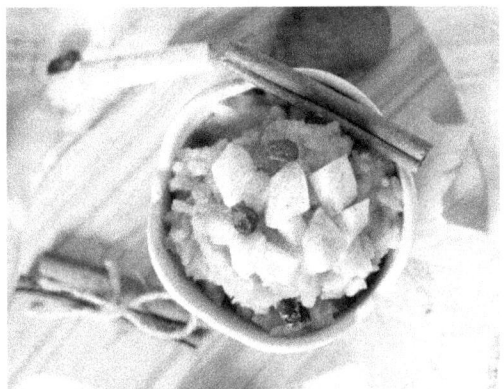

Prep Time: 15 minutes
Cook Time: 480 minutes
Total Time: 500 minutes
Servings: 12
Calories per serving: 150

Suitable for Vegetarians

Ingredients

- 3 cups coconut water
- 1 tsp. lime zest, finely grated
- 1¼ cups short grain brown rice
- 13.5 oz coconut milk
- 1 tbsp. vanilla extract
- ½ cup sugar
- 2 tbsp. butter, unsalted, cut into small pieces
- non-stick cooking spray
- ½ tsp. salt

Directions

- Lightly grease the bottom of your slow cooker with the non-stick cooking spray.
- Now, thoroughly combine the coconut milk with coconut water, vanilla, sugar, salt and 1½ cups water in the bowl of your slow cooker until the sugar is completely dissolved. Add the rice; give everything a good stir &cook for 4 hours on high heat settings.

- Uncover; give everything a good stir &let stand for a couple of minutes.
- Transfer everything together to a large-sized bowl & then stir in the butter. Let cool until warm, stirring frequently. Lastly stir in the finely grated lime zest. Feel free to add any of your favorite toppings such as raspberries, mango or pineapple.
- Serve warm or let cool and then serve.

Loaded Potato Soap

Prep Time: 15 minutes
Cook Time: 210 minutes (HIGH) or 360 minutes (LOW)
Total Time: 225 minutes (HIGH) or 375 minutes (LOW)
Servings: 4-6
Calories: 170

Ingredients
- 4-6 slices bacon, thick cut
- 1 tsp. ground pepper
- 6-7 cups potatoes; peeled and chopped into small chunks
- 1 cup heavy cream
- 3 cloves garlic, minced
- 1 cup onion, medium, chopped
- 3 cups chicken stock
- 1 cup Monterey Jack cheese, shredded, for garnish
- 1½ tsp. salt

Optional Ingredients
- Sour cream, green onions, croutons and fried onions, for garnish

Directions
- Add the entire vegetables to the bottom of your slow cooker. Pour in the chicken stock and then sprinkle with pepper and salt.
- Cover & cook on low heat settings for 6 hours or on high settings for approximately 3½ hours.

- In the meantime, over medium-high heat settings in a large skillet; cook the bacon. When done; drain and add the leftover bacon grease to the slow cooker; gently stir.
- Blend ½ of the potatoes with the heavy cream for a minute or two, until smooth and place it to the slow cooker as well.
- When ready to serve, garnish the soup with the cooked bacon and Monterey Jack cheese.

Dinner

Lemony Pork Roast

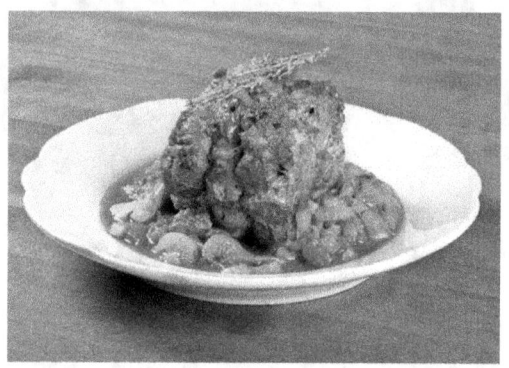

Prep Time: 5 minutes
Cook Time: 495 minutes
Total Time: 500 minutes
Servings: 8
Calories per serving: 317

Ingredients
- 1 garlic clove, minced
- 4 pork chops, boneless
- 1 onion, medium, sliced
- ½ tsp. ground cumin
- 1 red bell pepper, sliced
- ½ tsp. ground cinnamon
- 1 that apple, diced
- ½ cup coconut milk
- 1 cup squash, cubed
- 2 tbsp. parsley, fresh, chopped
- ½ cup chicken broth
- 2 tsp. olive oil
- ground black pepper to taste
- juice of 1 lemon, fresh

Directions
- Put everything together (except the Pork Chops) in a slow cooker and lastly add the pork chops over the top.
- Cover & cook for 8 hrs on low-heat settings.
- When done, transfer the pork carefully to a clean cutting board.
- Let rest for 10 minutes, until easy to handle and then slice into pieces.
- Transfer the vegetables and pork to the heated plates. Squeeze the lemon juice over the top.
- Serve & enjoy.

BBQ Pulled Pork

Prep Time: 10 minutes
Cook Time: 360 minutes (HIGH) or 480 minutes (LOW)
Total Time: 390 minutes (HIGH) or 510 minutes (LOW)
Servings: 8
Calories per serving: 323

Ingredients
- 1 pork shoulder roast (approximately 4 lbs.)
- 1 cup ketchup
- 1 cup barbeque sauce
- 2 cups celery, chopped
- 1 tsp. chilli powder
- ½ cup water
- 1 tsp. garlic powder
- 1 onion, medium, chopped
- salt& ground black pepper to taste

Directions
- Add celery together with the chilli powder, garlic powder, onion, ketchup, barbeque sauce, water, pepper and salt in the bottom of your slow cooker; give everything a good stir.
- Place the meat into the mixture; turn the pieces several times until evenly coated with the mixture.
- Cook for 5 hours on high heat setting or for 7 hours on low heat setting.
- Using two large forks; shred the meat and cook for an hour more.

- Serve warm and enjoy.

Chilli Beans and Sweet Potato

Prep Time: 5 minutes
Cook Time: 270 minutes (approx.)
Total Time: 275 minutes
Servings: 8
Calories per servings: 300.1

Suitable for Vegetarians

Ingredients
- 4 cloves garlic, minced
- 1 tbsp. chilli powder
- 1 ½ cups drained black beans
- 1 large sweet potato, cubed
- 3 small carrots, chopped
- 1 tsp. cocoa powder
- 28 oz. tomatoes, diced with juice
- 1 tbsp. cumin
- 2 tbsp. olive oil
- 1 cup water
- 2 tsp. sea salt

Directions
- Over moderate heat settings in a large saucepan; heat the oil and sauté garlic and onion. Add salt and the remaining vegetables.
- Put it the onion mixture as well.
- Transfer them to slow cooker.
- Cook on "high" for 6 hrs.
- Stir once and add 1 cup of Water.
- Cook again for 30 mins.
- Serve hot.

Chicken Stock

Prep Time: 10 minutes
Cook Time: 250 minutes
Total Time: 260 minutes
Servings: 5
Calories per serving: 246

Ingredients
- 4 pounds chicken legs
- 1 diced carrot
- 2 Thyme sprigs
- Bay leaf
- 1 chopped celery stalk
- 20 Peppercorns (whole)
- 1 clove garlic, crushed
- 6 Parsley sprigs
- 1 sliced onion
- 9 cups of Water

Directions
- Put everything together into the bottom of your slow cooker; give everything a good stir until evenly mixed.
- Close and cook for 4 hours on high-heat settings.
- Carefully remove the lid. Serve warm & enjoy.

Vegetable Pizza

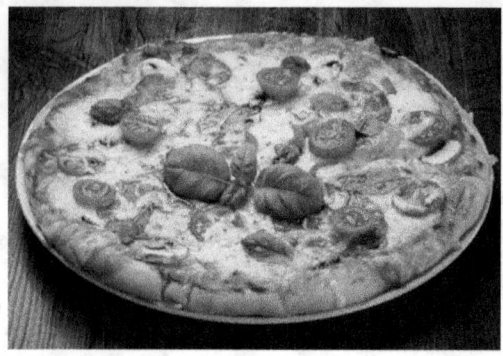

Prep Time: 15 minutes
Cook Time: 210 minutes
Total Time: 225 minutes
Servings: 8
Calories per servings: 174

Suitable for Vegetarians

Ingredients
- 1 cup part-skim mozzarella cheese, shredded
- 8 oz. pizza sauce
- 1 package refrigerated pizza dough (11 to 14 oz.)
- vegetable toppings such as broccoli florets, onions, peppers, mushrooms, halved cherry tomatoes, and artichoke hearts
- 14 oz. marinara
- Olive oil cooking spray

Directions
- Lightly coat the crock of your slow cooker with the olive oil cooking spray.
- Unroll the dough & then place them on the bottom of your slow cooker; spreading it out & pressing it with your fingers.
- Evenly spread the sauce over the crust.
- Sprinkle with approximately ¾ cup of cheese.
- Evenly scatter the vegetable toppings on top of the cheese.
- Sprinkle with the leftover cheese.

- Cover &cook until the crust around the edges begins to brown, from 2 to 2 1/2 hours on high heat settings.
- Carefully remove the lid and let stand for a couple of minutes.
- Carefully remove the pizza and cut into eight even-sized pieces.
- Serve warm and enjoy.

Chicken and Dumplings

Prep Time: 10 minutes
Cook Time: 360 minutes
Total Time: 370 minutes
Servings: 8
Calories per servings: 385

Ingredients
- 4 chicken breast halves, skinless, boneless
- 2 packages biscuit dough, refrigerated, torn into pieces (10 oz.)
- 1 onion, medium, diced finely
- 2 tbsp. Butter
- 11 oz. Condensed cream of chicken soup

Directions
- Place the meat together with soup, butter & onion into the bottom of your slow cooker & fill it with water enough to cover everything.
- Cover & cook on high heat settings for 5 to 6 hours.
- During the last 30 minutes of cooking, place the torn biscuit dough in the slow cooker. Cook for a couple of more minutes, until the dough is no longer raw in the middle.
- Serve warm and enjoy.

Tropical Chicken Dinner

Prep Time: 20 minutes
Cook Time: 360 minutes
Total Time: 380 minutes
Servings: 6
Calories per Servings: 361

Ingredients
- 4 chicken breast halves, skinless, boneless, cut into bite-sized pieces
- 1 tsp. ground ginger
- 4 sweet potatoes, peeled &cut into chunks
- 1 tsp. thyme, dried
- 20 oz. pineapple chunks, fresh
- 1 onion, medium, chopped
- 2 tbsp. Jamaican jerk seasoning
- 1 tbsp. lime zest, grated
- 2 tsp. Worcestershire sauce
- ½ cup raisins
- 1 tsp. ground cumin

Directions
- Place chicken together with onion &sweet potatoes into the bottom of your slow cooker.
- Mix the pineapple chunks together with raisins, Worcestershire sauce, ginger, lime zest, cumin and jerk seasoning in a large bowl until combined well.
- Pour the mixture on top of the chicken mixture and then sprinkle with thyme.
- Cover& cook for 6 hours on low heat settings, until the vegetables and chicken are tender.
- Serve warm and enjoy

Chicken Marrakesh

Prep Time: 25 minutes
Cook Time: 240 minutes
Total Time: 265 minutes
Servings: 8
Calories per servings: 290

Ingredients
- 2 carrots, large, peeled &diced
- 1 onion, sliced
- ½ tsp. ground turmeric
- 15 oz. garbanzo beans, rinsed
- ¼ tsp. ground cinnamon
- 2 pounds chicken breast halves, skinless, boneless, cut into 2" pieces
- ½ tsp. ground cumin
- 1 tsp. parsley, dried
- 2 sweet potatoes, large, peeled &diced
- ½ tsp. ground black pepper
- 14.5 oz. tomatoes, diced
- 1 tsp. salt

Optional Ingredients
- 2 garlic cloves, minced

Directions
- Place the sweet potatoes together with garlic, onion, chicken breast pieces, carrots, and garbanzo beans into the bottom of your slow cooker.
- Thoroughly combine the cumin with black pepper, cinnamon, parsley, turmeric, and salt in a large-sized bowl and then sprinkle the mixture over the vegetables and chicken.
- Add the tomatoes; give everything a good stir until evenly combined.
- Cover & cook for 4 hours on high heat settings, until the sauce has thickened &the sweet potatoes are tender.
- Serve warm and enjoy.

Chicken Tinga

Prep Time: 15 minutes
Cook Time: 165 minutes
Total Time: 180 minutes
Servings: 18 (half the ingredients for less)
Calories per serving: 131

Ingredients
- 15 oz. tomato sauce
- 1 onion, medium, chopped
- 3/4 chorizo sausage (approximately 1 lb.)
- 7 ounce chipotle chilli peppers in adobo sauce, chopped & seeded
- 1 tsp. ground oregano
- 4 chicken breast halves, skinless, boneless
- 1 tsp. chilli powder
- 2 jalapeno peppers, fresh, seeded &chopped
- 1 tsp. ground cumin
- 2 garlic cloves, minced
- ¼ tsp. red pepper flakes

Directions
- Add the chicken pieces together with cumin, tomato sauce, onion, jalapeno peppers, chipotle chilli peppers in adobo sauce, garlic, oregano, red pepper flakes and chilli powder in the bottom of your slow cooker; give everything a good stir until evenly mixed.
- Cook for 2 hours on low heat settings, until the chicken is no longer pink in the middle.
- Remove the cooked chicken from slow cooker and using 2 large forks; shred the meat.
- Over medium-high heat settings in a large skillet; cook &stir the chorizo sausage for a couple of minutes, until browned &crumbly then drain it &discard the grease; add chorizo into the chicken mixture; give everything a good stir.
- Cook for 45 minutes to 55 minutes on low heat settings.

Chicken Stroganoff

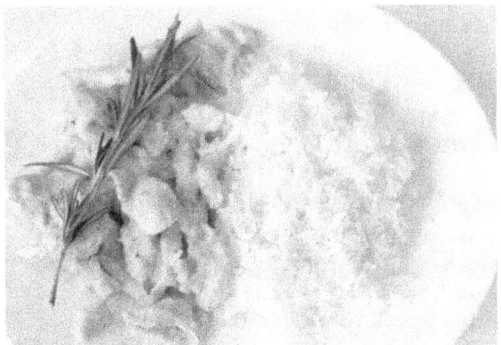

Prep Time: 10 minutes
Cook Time: 360 minutes
Total Time: 370 minutes
Servings: 4
Calories per servings: 256

Ingredients
- 4 chicken breast halves, skinless, boneless, cubed
- 1 package Italian-style salad dressing mix, dry (7 Oz.)
- 10.75 oz. condensed cream of chicken soup
- ⅛ cup butter
- 1 package cream cheese (8 Oz.)

Directions
- Put chicken pieces together with butter & dressing mix into the bottom of your slow cooker; mix well &cook for 5 to 6 hours on low heat settings.
- Add the soup and cream cheese; give everything a good stir until evenly mixed and cook until heated through and warm, for 30 more minutes on high heat settings.

Eggplant Parmesan

Prep Time: 30 minutes

Cook Time: 300 minutes
Total Time: 330 minutes
Servings: 8
Calories per servings: 401

Ingredients
- 4 eggplants, peeled &cut into ½" slices
- 1/3 cup bread crumbs, seasoned
- 2 eggs, large
- 1 package mozzarella cheese, sliced (16 oz.)
- 3 tbsp. all-purpose flour
- 1 jar prepared marinara sauce (32 oz.)
- ½ cup parmesan cheese, grated
- 1 cup extra-virgin olive oil, or to taste
- 1/3 cup water
- 1 tbsp. salt, or to taste

Directions
- Working in layers; place slices of eggplant in a bowl, preferably large-sized and then sprinkle each layer with some salt. Let stand for half an hour; and then rinse and place them on paper towels to drain.
- Over medium heat settings in a large skillet; heat the olive oil. Whisk eggs with flour and water until completely smooth.
- Work in batches and dip the eggplant slices into the batter &fry in the hot oil for a couple of minutes, until golden brown.
- Now, in a large-sized bowl; mix the seasoned bread crumbs with the Parmesan cheese. Place ¼ of the eggplant slices into the slow cooker &top with ¼ of the crumbs, ¼ of the mozzarella cheese & ¼ of the marinara sauce. Repeat these layers a couple of more times.
- Cover &cook for 4 to 5 hours on low heat settings, until flavours have blended and tender.

South-western Vegetarian Dinner

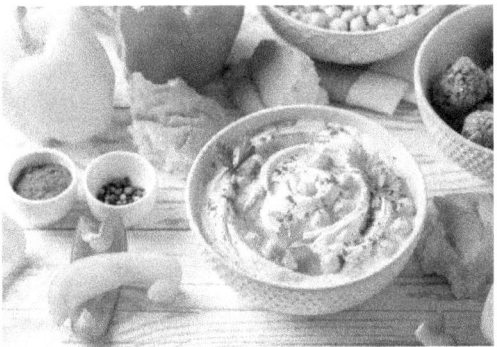

Prep Time: 5 minutes
Cook Time: 150 minutes
Total Time: 155 minutes
Servings: 6
Calories per serving: 342

Suitable for Vegetarians

Ingredients
- 28 oz. tomatoes, diced
- ½ cup black-eyed peas, dried, soaked for overnight
- 10 oz. sweet corn
- 1 onion, chopped
- garlic cloves, chopped
- 2 cups rice, cooked
- 1 green bell pepper, diced
- ½ cup cheddar cheese, shredded
- 2 tsp. ground cumin
- ¼ cup chilli powder

Directions
- Drain & thoroughly rinse the black-eyed peas.
- Now, place the peas together with garlic, onion, green pepper, tomatoes and corn into the bottom of your slow cooker.
- Season with cumin & chilli powder; give everything a good stir until blended well.
- Cover &cook for 2 hours on high heat settings.

- Stir in the rice & cheese. Continue cooking for 30 more minutes.
- Serve warm and enjoy.

Cacciatore Chicken

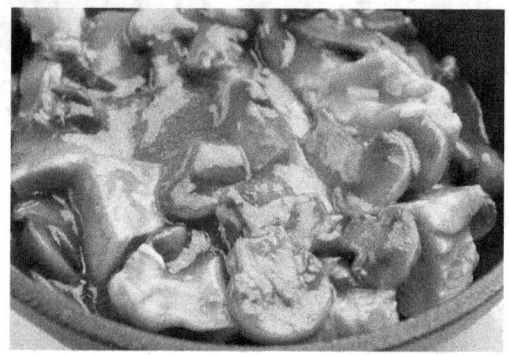

Prep Time: 15 minutes
Cook Time: 265 minutes
Total Time: 280 minutes
Servings: 6
Calories per serving: 277

Ingredients
- 1/3 cup all-purpose flour
- 2 sliced onions
- 1 sliced green pepper
- 6 oz. mushroom
- ½ tsp. oregano, dried
- 14 oz. tomatoes, diced
- ¼ tsp. basil, dried
- 2 cloves garlic, minced
- ½ cup parmesan, shredded
- 2 tbsp. canola oil
- salt

Directions

- Coat the chicken pieces with the flour in a large-sized plastic bag.
- Now, brown the coated chicken pieces over moderate heat settings in a large-sized skillet.
- Transfer it to the slow cooker.
- Place the remaining ingredients over the chicken.
- Cook them on "low" for 4 hrs.
- Serve hot after garnishing with Parmesan.

Pepper Steak

Prep Time: 20 minutes
Cook Time: 240 minutes (HIGH) or 420 minutes (LOW) (approx.)
Total Time: 260 minutes (HIGH) or 440 minutes (LOW) (approx.)
Servings: 6
Calories per serving: 301

Ingredients
- 2 pounds beef sirloin, cut into 2 inch strips
- 1 tbsp. corn-starch
- 3 tbsp. vegetable oil
- 1 beef bouillon, cubed
- 2 green bell peppers, large, chopped roughly
- ½ cup onion, chopped
- 1 tsp. white sugar
- garlic powder, to taste
- ¼ cup hot water
- 3 tbsp. soy sauce

Directions
- Sprinkle the sirloin strips with garlic powder.
- Over medium heat settings in a large skillet; heat the vegetable oil & cook the seasoned beef strips until brown, for a couple of minutes.
- Transfer the cooked beef strips to the bottom of your slow cooker.

- Mix the bouillon cube with hot water; mix well until completely dissolved and then add the corn-starch; mix until dissolved as well.
- Pour the mixture over the meat into the slow cooker and then stir in the stewed tomatoes, onion, sugar, green peppers, soy sauce and salt.
- Cover & cook for 3 to 4 hours on high heat setting or for 6 to 8 hours on low heat settings.
- Serve warm and enjoy.

Vegetarian Chilli

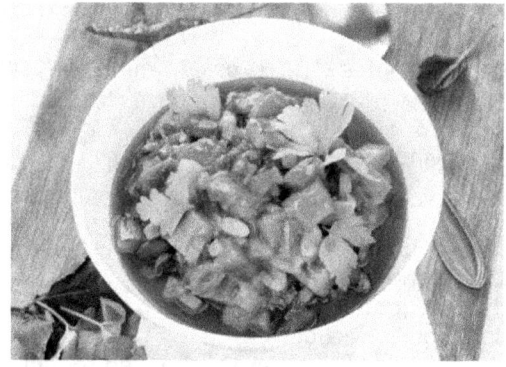

Prep Time: 10 minutes
Cook Time: 120 minutes
Total Time: 130 minutes
Servings: 8
Calories per serving: 260

Suitable for Vegetarians

Ingredients
- 19 oz. black bean soup
- 15 oz. kidney beans, rinsed
- 1 onion, chopped
- 15 oz. whole kernel corn

- 1 green bell pepper, chopped
- 2 stalks celery, chopped
- 1 tbsp. chilli powder, or to taste
- 14.5 oz. tomatoes, chopped
- 1 tbsp. parsley, dried
- 2 garlic cloves, chopped
- 1 tbsp. oregano, dried
- 15 oz. garbanzo beans, rinsed
- 1 tbsp. basil, dried

Directions
- Thoroughly mix the black bean soup with kidney beans, tomatoes, baked beans, garbanzo beans, onion, corn, celery and bell pepper into the bottom of your slow cooker.
- Season with chilli powder, garlic, parsley, basil and oregano.
- Cook on high heat settings for 2 hours.
- Serve warm and enjoy.

Pork and Sauerkraut with Apples

Prep Time: 10 minutes
Cook Time: 240 minutes (HIGH) or 420 minutes (LOW)
Total Time: 250 minutes (HIGH) or 430 minutes (LOW)
Servings: 6
Calories per serving: 400

Ingredients
- 6 pork chops, thick-cut
- 1 quart sauerkraut
- 4 tart apples, peeled &sliced
- ½ teaspoon fennel seed, or to taste
- 1 onion, large, sliced
- water to cover

Directions
- Over medium-high heat settings in a large skillet; cook the pork chops for a couple of minutes until brown per side; place them on paper towels to drain.

- Arrange the apples &onion in the bottom of your slow cooker and then top them with the cooked pork chops. Pour in the water enough to cover the bottom.
- Cook for 6 hours on low heat settings or for 3 hours on high-heat settings.
- Add the fennel seed and sauerkraut to pork chop mixture. Cook for an hour more.
- Serve warm and enjoy.

Yummy Chuck Roast

Prep Time: 10 minutes
Cook Time: 530 minutes
Total Time: 540
Servings: 8
Calories per serving: 501

Ingredients
- 2 tbsp. Dill Weed, chopped
- 1 pound halved mushrooms
- 2 pounds beef chuck roast
- 1 chopped onion
- 2 tbsp. corn-starch
- ½ cup sour crème, low-fat
- 2 tbsp. dijon mustard
- black pepper

Directions
- Over moderate heat settings in your slow cooker; sauté the mushrooms, onion and beef; sprinkle with the pepper and salt to taste.
- Close and cook on "low" for 8 hrs. Stir when done.
- In a bowl, mix corn-starch with 2 cups of water.
- Boil starch mixture in a pan for 1 min.
- When beef is done, add starch mixture and the rest of the ingredients in the slow cooker.
- Before serving, heat the plates.
- Serve the beef on the heated plates after garnishing with dill.

Cabbage Rolls

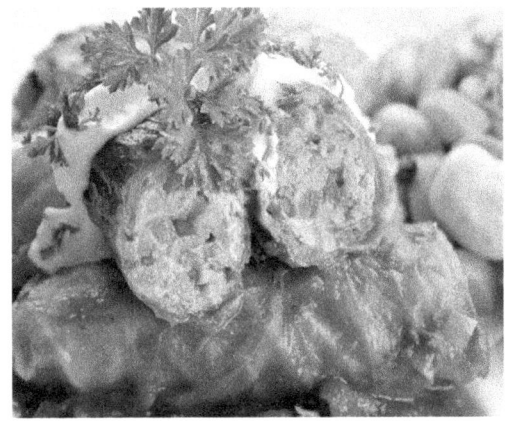

Prep Time: 30 minutes
Cook Time: 510 minutes
Total Time: 540 minutes
Servings: 6
Calories per serving: 246

Ingredients
- 1 beaten egg, large
- 12 leaves, cabbage
- 1 tbsp. brown sugar
- ¼ cup milk
- 1 cup white rice, cooked
- ¼ cup onion, minced
- 1 lb. ground beef, extra-lean
- 1¼ tsp. ground black pepper
- 1 tbsp. lemon juice, fresh
- 8 oz. tomato sauce
- 1 tsp. Worcestershire sauce
- 1¼ tsp. salt

Directions
- Fill a large pot with water and bring it to a boil over moderate heat settings.

- Boil the cabbage leaves for a couple of minutes and then drain.
- Combine the cooked rice together with milk, egg, ground beef, onion, pepper and salt in a large-sized bowl.
- Place approximately ¼ cup of the meat mixture in middle of each cabbage leaf; roll up and tucking the ends in.
- Place the rolls in your slow cooker.
- Mix tomato sauce together with lemon juice, brown sugar & Worcestershire sauce in a small-sized bowl and pour the mixture on top of the cabbage rolls.
- Cover & cook for 8 to 9 hours on Low heat settings.
- Serve warm and enjoy.

Beer Braised Chicken

Prep Time: 5 minutes
Cook Time: 240 minutes (HIGH) or 480minutes (LOW)
Total Time: 245 minutes (HIGH) or 485minutes (LOW)
Servings: 8
Calories per serving: 318

Ingredients
- 4 boneless, skinless chicken breasts
- ¼ cup water mixed with 2 tbsp. corn-starch
- 2 tbsp. hot sauce
- 1 oz. diced tomatoes
- 2 red peppers, chopped
- 1 onion, finely chopped
- 2 andouille sausage links quartered
- 1 tsp. smoked paprika
- 4 diced green chillies
- 1 tbsp. chilli powder
- ½ tsp. cayenne pepper
- 2 tsp. dried thyme
- cooked brown or white rice for serving
- 1 oz. pumpkin beer
- Parsley, fresh for garnish
- ¼ tsp. each pepper & salt

Directions

- Scatter the onions in the bottom of the slow cooker and then add the Andouille sausage, green chillies, red peppers, tomatoes, chilli powder, hot sauce, thyme, paprika, cayenne, pepper and salt.
- Add the chicken pieces & beer; make sure you submerge the chicken pieces in the mixture.
- Cook for 7 to 8 hours on low heat settings or for 4 hours on high heat settings.
- During the last 30 minutes of your cooking, add the corn-starch mixture; give everything a good stir until evenly combined.
- Cook for 20 to 30 more minutes on high heat settings, until the sauce thickens.
- Serve with rice & garnish your recipe with fresh parsley.

Tarragon Lamb Shanks with Cannellini Beans

Prep Time: 5 minutes
Cook Time: 600 minutes
Total Time: 605 minutes
Servings: 12
Calories per serving: 353

Ingredients
- 4 lamb shanks (1½ lbs.); trim the fat
- 1 cup onion, chopped
- 28 oz. tomatoes, diced
- 1½ cups carrot, peeled, diced
- 19 oz. cannellini beans, rinsed
- ¾ cup celery, chopped
- 2 cloves garlic, sliced thinly
- ¼ tsp. freshly ground black pepper
- 2 tsp. tarragon, dried
- ½ tsp. salt

Directions

- Place the carrot together with beans, onion, tomato and garlic in the bottom of your slow cooker; give everything a good stir until evenly mixed.
- Place the lamb shanks over the bean mixture and then sprinkle with tarragon, pepper & salt.
- Pour the tomatoes on top of the lamb.
- Cover &cook for an hour on high heat settings.
- Decrease the heat settings to low & cook until the lamb is very tender, for 9 hours.
- Carefully remove the lamb shanks from your slow cooker.
- Using a sieve or colander; pour the bean mixture over a bowl; reserving the liquid.
- Let the liquid stand for a couple of minutes and skim the fat from surface of liquid.
- Return the bean mixture to the liquid.
- Remove the lamb from bones; discarding the bones.
- Serve lamb with rice, bean mixture & garnish with fresh parsley.

Pesto Lasagne with Spinach and Mushrooms

Prep Time: 10 minutes
Cook Time: 300 minutes
Total Time: 305 minutes
Servings: 8
Calories per serving: 398

Ingredients
- 4 cups torn spinach
- ¾ cup part-skim mozzarella cheese, shredded
- 1 bottle basil-tomato pasta sauce, fat-free (25.5 oz.)
- 2 cups cremini mushrooms, sliced
- ¾ cup Parmesan cheese, fresh, grated, divided
- 12 lasagna noodles, precooked
- ¾ cup provolone cheese, shredded
- 15 oz. Ricotta cheese, fat-free
- ½ cup commercial pesto

- 8 oz. tomato sauce
- 1 lightly beaten egg, large
- cooking spray

Directions
- Place the spinach in a vegetable steamer; cover & steam the spinach until the spinach wilts, for a couple of minutes and then drain; squeezing it dry and then chop it coarsely.
- Combine spinach together with pesto and mushrooms in a medium-sized bowl; give everything a good stir until evenly combined; set aside.
- Now, in a medium-sized bowl; combine the mozzarella with ricotta, provolone & beaten egg; give everything a good stir until combined well.
- Stir in approximately ¼ cup of the Parmesan cheese; set aside.
- Combine the tomato sauce &the pasta sauce in a medium-sized bowl.
- Spread approximately 1 cup of the pasta sauce mixture into the bottom of your slow cooker lightly coated with the cooking spray, then arrange 3 noodles on top of the pasta sauce mixture; top with approximately 1 cup of spinach mixture and 1 cup of cheese mixture.
- Repeat these layers; ending with the spinach mixture.
- Arrange 3 noodles on top of the spinach mixture& then top with the leftover 1 cup of the pasta sauce mixture and 1 cup of cheese mixture.
- Place the leftover 3 noodles on top of the sauce mixture; spreading the leftover sauce mixture on top of the noodles.
- Sprinkle the leftover Parmesan cheese; cover &cook until done, for 5 hours on low heat settings.
- Serve and enjoy.

Cassoulet

Prep Time: 10 minutes
Cook Time: 300 minutes
Total Time: 310 minutes
Servings: 8
Calories per serving: 219

Ingredients
- 1 lb. lean pork loin roast, boneless, trimmed &cut into 1" cubes
- 2 cups onion, chopped
- 30 oz. great northern beans, rinsed
- 1 tsp. thyme, dried
- 8 tsp. parmesan cheese, fresh &shredded finely
- 3 cloves garlic, minced
- 14.5 oz. tomatoes, diced
- ½ tsp. rosemary, dried
- 2 slices bacon
- 8 tsp. flat-leaf parsley, fresh, chopped
- ½ tsp. each freshly ground black pepper and salt

Directions
- Over medium-high heat settings in a large skillet; cook the bacon slices until crispy.
- Remove the bacon from pan and then crumble.
- Add thyme, onion, garlic and rosemary to the drippings in the pan and sauté until tender, for a couple of minutes.
- Stir in the crumbled bacon, tomatoes, pepper and salt; bring everything together to a boil. Once boiling, remove from heat.
- Place ½ of the beans in a large-sized bowl; using a potato masher, mash until chunky.
- Add the leftover beans & pork; give everything a good stir.
- Place ½ of bean mixture in a slow cooker and then top with ½ of tomato mixture.
- Repeat these layers; cover &cook for 5 hours on low heat settings.
- Ladle into bowls and then sprinkle with Parmesan cheese & parsley.

Creamy Tortellini Soup

Prep Time: 5 minutes
Cook Time: 420 minutes
Total Time: 425 minutes
Servings: 6

Calories per serving: 253.5

Ingredients
- 1 lb. ground beef, cooked & browned
- 24 oz. jar spaghetti sauce
- 8 oz. cream cheese, cut into 1" cubes
- ¼ cup onion, diced
- 4 cups beef broth
- 3-4 garlic cloves, minced
- ½ cup carrots, diced
- 16 oz. cheese tortellini, refrigerated
- 4 cups spinach leaves, fresh, packed loosely
- 8 oz. sliced mushrooms, fresh
- 2 cups water

Directions
- Combine the browned beef together with spaghetti sauce, garlic, onions, carrots, beef broth, mushrooms, cream cheese, spinach and water in a slow cooker; give everything a good stir.
- Cook for 7 hours on low heat settings.
- Whisk well and ensure there are no chunks of the cream cheese and then stir in the tortellini. Cover & cook until hot and tender, for 20 to 30 more minutes.
- Serve hot & enjoy.

Shio Ramen and Chilli Oil

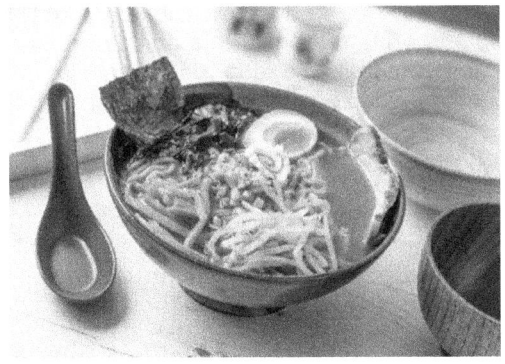

Prep Time: 5 minutes
Cook Time: 480 minutes
Total Time: 485 minutes
Servings: 6
Calories per serving: 160

Suitable for Vegetarians

Ingredients
- 4 carrots, cut into ½" chunks
- 1 cup shitake mushrooms, sliced
- 2 cloves garlic, minced
- 1 large onion, diced
- 8 cups water
- 1 tbsp. ginger, fresh &minced
- Ramen Noodles
- 1 tsp. salt

Chilli Oil Ingredients
- 1 tsp. red pepper flakes
- ½ cup olive oil

Directions
- Combine shitake mushrooms together with carrot chunks, onion chunks, garlic, ginger, water and salt in a large slow cooker.
- Cook for 8 hours on high heat settings.
- Now, combine the red pepper flakes and olive oil in a small saucepan, cook for a couple of minutes over medium-low heat settings.
- Remove from heat; strain & let cool and then set aside.
- When ready, strain the slow cooker contents into a large saucepan and bring the broth to a boil over moderate heat settings & then add in the ramen noodles.
- Cook for a couple of more minutes, until the noodles are done.
- Remove the noodles from the broth &put them in a serving bowl. Top with your favorite add-ins such as bamboo shoots, shitake mushrooms, baby bok-Choy, corn, scallions, boiled egg, bean sprouts or chicken.
- When ready, spoon the broth into individual bowls and then drizzle with the chilli oil.
- Serve hot& enjoy.

Red Pepper, Feta and Kale Frittata

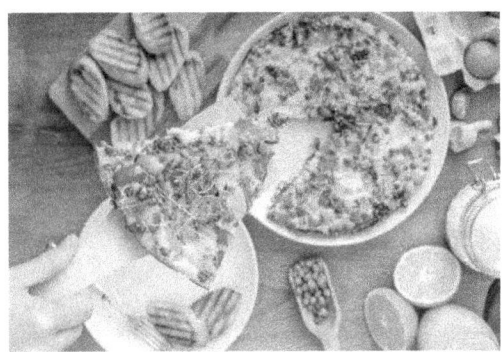

Prep Time: 5 minutes
Cook Time: 150 minutes
Total Time: 155 minutes
Servings: 6-8
Calories per serving: 270

Suitable for Vegetarians

Ingredients
- 8 eggs, well beaten
- 5 oz. Baby kale; washed & spin dry, or place it on paper towel to dry
- ¼ cup green onion, sliced
- 6 oz. Red pepper, roasted, diced
- rresh-ground black pepper, to taste
- 4-5 oz. Feta, crumbled
- 1 - 2 tsp. Olive oil
- ½ tsp. all-purpose seasoning
- Olive Oil Cooking Spray

Optional Ingredients
- Sour cream, low-fat

Directions
- Heat the oil over high-heat settings in a slow cooker.

- When hot, sauté the kale until softened; leaving it for a couple of minutes in the slow cooker.
- Drain the red peppers & then chop into fairly small pieces.
- Add the sliced green onion and chopped red pepper to the slow cooker.
- Beat the eggs and then transfer it over the ingredients in the slow cooker; give everything a good stir until the ingredients are combined well.
- Season with black pepper and all-purpose seasoning; then sprinkle with the Feta.
- Cook for 2 to 3 hours on low heat settings or until the cheese is completely melted and frittata is completely set.
- Serve hot with a dollop of sour cream & enjoy.

Ropa Vieja

Prep Time: 15 minutes
Cook Time: 480 minutes
Total Time: 495 minutes
Servings: 4
Calories per serving: 464

Ingredients
- 1½ lbs. flank steak or skirt steak
- 3 tbsp. ketchup
- 1½ tsp. ground cumin
- 15 oz. tomatoes, crushed
- 1 tbsp. grapple cider vinegar
- 2 garlic cloves, minced
- 1 onion, small, sliced thinly
- 2 bell peppers (1 green, 1 red), sliced into ½" thick
- 1 jalapeno pepper, sliced thinly (with seeds)
- white rice, cooked, for serving
- 3 tbsp. pimiento-stuffed green olives, chopped, plus 1 tbsp. brine from jar
- salt to taste

Directions

- Place tomatoes together with cumin, garlic, vinegar, ketchup, ¾ tsp. Salt and jalapeno into the bottom of your slow cooker; give everything a good stir until evenly combined.
- Add the steak, onion and bell peppers; toss well until coated well. Cover & cook for 8 hours on low heat settings, undisturbed.
- Uncover & skim any excess fat off.
- Using two forks; shred the meat coarsely and then stir in the olive brine and olives.
- Serve over some cooked rice & enjoy.

Turkey Mole Tacos

Prep Time: 15 minutes
Cook Time: 480 minutes
Total Time: 495 minutes
Servings: 6
Calories per serving: 464

Ingredients
- 1 bone-in turkey breast, skinless (approximately 2½ lbs.)
- 15 oz. Tomatoes, diced
- 2 tsp. Cocoa powder, unsweetened
- 1 green bell pepper, finely chopped
- 4 chopped scallions, plus more for topping
- ¼ cup fresh cilantro, chopped roughly, plus more for topping
- 2 carrots, large, cut into ½" pieces
- 1½ tbsp. Soy sauce, low-sodium
- 2 tbsp. Peanut butter
- 18 corn tortillas
- 1 tbsp. Anchor-chilli powder
- ½ tsp. Ground cinnamon or Chinese five-spice powder

Directions

- Combine tomatoes together with soy sauce, cilantro, bell pepper, carrots, peanut butter, scallions, chilli powder, ground cinnamon or Chinese five-spice powder and cocoa powder in a slow cooker; give everything a good stir until evenly combined.
- Add the turkey; turning the meat several times to coat well with the mixture.
- Cover & cook for 8 hours on low heat settings.
- Remove the turkey & transfer it to a large plate; shred it using two large forks & get rid of the bone.
- Place the shredded meat to the slow cooker again; stir well to coat.
- Warm the tortillas in the microwave.
- Serve the turkey in the tortillas &top with more scallions and cilantro.

Chicken and Vegetable Soup

Prep Time: 15 minutes
Cook Time: 480 minutes
Total Time: 495 minutes
Servings: 8
Calories per serving: 146

Ingredients
- 3 skin-on chicken breasts, bone-in, skinned &excess fat trimmed (approximately 1½ lbs.)
- ½ cup fresh dill fronds, loosely packed, chopped
- 3 carrots, medium, sliced into ¼" thick rounds
- 1 cup peas, frozen
- 2 celery stalks, peeled &sliced finely
- 1 onion, medium, chopped
- 4 cups chicken broth, low-sodium
- 1 piece Parmesan rind (approximately 2")
- 3 parsnips, medium, sliced into ¼" thick half-moon shapes
- Freshly ground black pepper-and-salt, to taste
- 1 tsp. Yellow curry powder
- Parmesan, grated and lemon for serving

Directions
- Combine chicken breasts together with carrots, parsnips, curry powder, onions, celery, Parmesan rind, 2 cups water, chicken broth, a few grinds of black pepper & 1 tsp. Salt in the insert of your slow cooker.
- Cook for 8 hours on low heat settings.
- Remove the chicken breasts; set aside and let cool until easy to handle.
- When cool, shred the meat using two large forks & discard the bones and then add them to the soup again; add the dill and peas.
- Season with pepper and salt.
- Serve in individual soup bowls with a squeeze of lemon &a sprinkle of Parmesan.

French Dip Sandwiches

Prep Time: 20 minutes
Cook Time: 140 minutes
Total Time: 165 minutes
Servings: 6-8
Calories per serving: 373

Ingredients
- 3 scallions, roughly chopped (light green and white parts only)
- 1 beef eye round roast, trim any excess fat (approximately 2½ lbs.)
- 2 tsp. thyme, fresh
- 1 garlic clove, crushed
- 2 tbsp. Worcestershire sauce
- ¼ tsp. ground allspice
- 2 carrots, sliced into 1" thick pieces
- ¼ tsp. celery seeds
- 6 to 8 Kaiser rolls, split &warmed
- freshly ground pepper-and-salt, to taste
- 1 cube beef bouillon
- spicy mustard and/or creamy horseradish, for serving

Directions

- Prepare the paste: Pulse the garlic together with thyme, scallions, the celery seeds, 1 tsp. Of each pepper & salt and the allspice in a food processor.
- Using a paring knife; pierce the roast completely and then rub the meat with the spice paste.
- To help keep its shape; tie the roast with the kitchen twine.
- Spread the carrots in a slow cooker & then set the roast over the top.
- Combine the Worcestershire sauce together with bouillon cube and 1½ cups of water in a microwave-safe bowl; microwave for a couple of minutes, until hot and then add the mixture to the slow cooker.
- Cover &cook for 2 hours on low heat settings.
- Transfer the cooked meat to a clean cutting board & cover with foil; let rest for a couple of minutes.
- Skim the excess fat off from the cooking liquid.
- Remove the twine & then thinly slice the meat.
- Spoon some of the cooking liquid over the cut sides of each roll; sandwich with meat, mustard and/or horseradish.
- Serve with more of the cooking liquid and enjoy.

Chicken Tortilla Soup

Prep Time: 20 minutes
Cook Time: 480 minutes
Total Time: 500 minutes
Servings: 4
Calories per serving: 224

Ingredients

- 1¼ lb. bone-in chicken thighs, skinless
- 14.5 oz. tomatoes, diced
- ½ red bell pepper, chopped
- 1 clove garlic, chopped
- 2 oz. chicken stock
- 1 onion, small, chopped
- 4 oz. green chillies, chopped
- 1 tsp. oregano, dried
- 8 oz. tomato sauce

- 1 tsp. chilli powder
- 2½ tbsp. chopped fresh cilantro, for serving
- sour cream, sliced jalapeños and tortilla chips, for serving
- ¾ tsp. ground cumin
- freshly ground black pepper & salt to taste

Directions
- Add chicken together with diced tomatoes, bell pepper, onion, stock, garlic, chilli powder, chillies, tomato sauce, cumin and oregano into the bottom of your slow cooker.
- Season with pepper and salt to taste.
- Cover & cook for 7 to 8 hours on low heat settings, until the chicken is cooked through.
- Remove the chicken; get rid of the bones & then shred the meat using two large forks.
- Place the shredded meat to the slow cooker again; add the cilantro; give everything a good stir.
- Top with sour cream, jalapeños, fresh cilantro and with some tortilla chips on side. Serve & enjoy.

Tex-Mex Casserole

Prep Time: 30 minutes
Cook Time: 255 minutes
Total Time: 285 minutes
Servings: 4-6
Calories per serving: 443

Suitable for Vegetarians

Ingredients
- 2 avocados, sliced
- ½ cup cilantro, fresh, chopped, plus more for topping
- 2 tsp. ground cumin
- 1 tsp. anchor chilli powder
- 2 poblano chilli peppers, seeded &chopped
- 1 jar spicy salsa (16 oz.)
- 30 oz. pinto beans, refried
- 2 cups fire-roasted corn, frozen

- 10 oz. green chillies and tomatoes, diced
- 2 cups cheddar cheese, shredded
- 18 to 20 corn tostada shells
- 2 cups Muenster cheese, shredded

Directions
- Combine the frozen corn together with refried beans, ¼ cup cilantro, poblanos, chilli powder and cumin in a large-sized bowl.
- Combine the tomatoes with salsa and a leftover ¼ cup of cilantro in a separate bowl, preferably medium-sized.
- Toss the Muenster and cheddar cheese in a separate bowl; set aside.
- Spread approximately ½ cup of the salsa mixture in a slow cooker, preferably in a thin layer.
- Top with approximately 6 of the tostada shells, breaking them as required and make sure it covers the bottom.
- Spread ½ of the bean mixture on top of the tostada shells and then sprinkle 1 cup of the salsa mixture &1½ cups of the cheese mixture.
- Repeat these layers and top with the leftover tostadas, salsa and cheese.
- Cover &cook for 4 hours on low heat settings.
- Uncover &let stand for a couple of minutes.
- Serve with sliced avocados& fresh cilantro.

Moroccan Chicken and Squash

Prep Time: 15 minutes
Cook Time: 240 minutes
Total Time: 255 minutes
Servings: 4
Calories per serving: 292

Ingredients
- 4 bone-in chicken legs, skin-on with drumsticks & thighs attached
- 8 oz. butternut squash, peeled & cut into large-sized chunks
- ½ cup golden raisins

- 3 cups chicken broth, low-sodium
- 1 leek (light green and white parts only), chopped
- ½ tsp. turmeric
- 1 turnip, large, peeled & cut into large chunks
- freshly ground pepper & salt taste
- 1 tsp. ground cumin
- juice & zest of 1 lemon, grated
- 2 tbsp. tomato paste
- couscous, for serving
- 1 tsp. ground coriander
- fresh cilantro, for topping

Directions
- Thoroughly mix the squash with turnip, raisins and leek in a slow cooker.
- Season the chicken with pepper and salt; place them over the vegetables.
- Now, in a large bowl; whisk the tomato paste together with chicken broth, coriander, cumin, lemon zest and juice, turmeric &1 tsp. salt.
- Pour the mixture on top of the vegetables and chicken.
- Cover &cook for 4 hours on high heat settings.
- Serve the vegetables and chicken with couscous &top with fresh cilantro.

Salmon with Cilantro and Lime

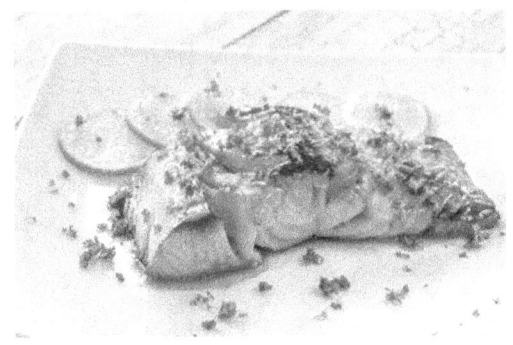

Prep Time: 15 minutes
Cook Time: 150 minutes
Total Time: 165 minutes
Servings: 4
Calories per serving: 212

Suitable for Vegetarians

Ingredients
- 4 salmon fillets
- 2½ tbsp. lime juice, freshly squeezed
- ¾ cup cilantro with stems removed, chopped
- 1 tbsp. olive oil
- 2 garlic cloves, pressed or finely chopped
- ¼ tsp. salt

Directions
- Lightly coat the bottom of your slow cooker with the olive oil.
- Arrange the fillets into the slow cooker, preferably skin side down.
- Add garlic together with cilantro, olive oil, lime juice &salt in a small bowl, mix well and then pour the mixture on top of the salmon fillets.
- Cover and cook for 1½ hours on high heat settings. Serve immediately& enjoy.

Steak Roulade with Provolone

Prep Time: 25 minutes
Cook Time: 425 minutes
Total Time: 450 minutes
Servings: 6
Calories per serving: 279

Ingredients
- 28 oz. Whole San Marzano tomatoes, crushed by hand
- ½ tsp. Red pepper flakes
- 1 cup panko bread crumbs
- ½ tsp. Sugar

- 1 small bunch basil, torn (approximately 10 leaves)
- 12 oz. Tomato paste
- 1⅔ cups provolone cheese, grated
- ½ cup pecorino Romano cheese, grated (approximately 2 ounces)
- 3 garlic cloves, small, minced
- 1 cup parsley, fresh, lightly packed
- ¼ cup chopped walnuts or pine nuts
- Polenta, for serving
- 1 flank steak (1½-1¾ lbs.)
- Freshly ground pepper & salt to taste
- ⅓ cup golden raisins

Directions

- Combine the tomato paste together with 2 cups hot water in a slow cooker.
- Add the red pepper flakes, crushed tomatoes, basil and sugar; give everything a good stir until evenly combined.
- Cover &cook on high settings and prepare the meat.
- Slice the steak horizontally in half; leaving 1 long side attached.
- Place them among 2 plastic wrap pieces &pound it until it's approximately ¼" thick.
- Remove the plastic &season the steak with pepper and salt.
- Evenly scatter the provolone on top of the steak and then top with the raisins, garlic, pecorino, breadcrumbs, pine nuts &parsley.
- Beginning with a long side, roll up the steak tightly just like a jelly roll.
- Secure with twine in different spots.
- Transfer to the slow cooker; cover and cook on low heat settings for 7 hours.
- Remove the meat & place on a clean cutting board; let it rest for a couple of minutes.
- Remove the twine & then slice into 1" thick.
- Top with some additional sauce from the slow cooker and serve with polenta.

Ham with Barbeque Beans

Prep Time: 10 minutes
Cook Time: 480 minutes
Total Time: 480 minutes
Servings: 8-10
Calories per serving: 214

Ingredients
- 1 bone-in picnic ham (4-7 lbs.)
- ½ cup ketchup
- 1 tsp. Apple cider vinegar
- ¼ cup packed dark brown sugar
- 1 onion, small, chopped finely
- ¼ cup maple syrup
- 2 tsp. Worcestershire sauce
- 1½ tbsp. molasses
- 2 tbsp. yellow mustard
- 1 lb. navy beans, dried, picked over
- freshly ground pepper, to taste

Directions
- Combine beans together with onion, Worcestershire sauce, maple syrup, brown sugar, ketchup, molasses, mustard, vinegar, ¼ tsp. Pepper and 3 cups water in a slow cooker.
- Place the ham over the top; cover &cook for 8 hours on high heat settings.
- Transfer the ham to a large platter &skim the excess fat from the beans off.
- Slice the ham into pieces & serve with beans.

Salmon Chowder with Dill

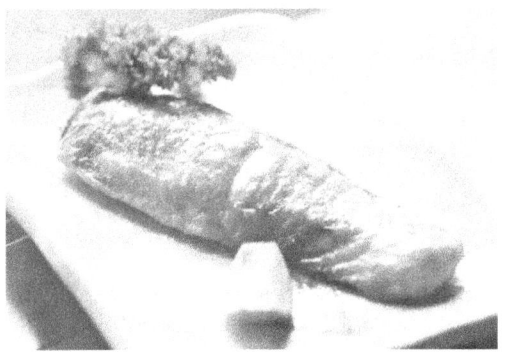

Prep Time: 20 minutes
Cook Time: 240 minutes
Total Time: 260 minutes
Servings: 4
Calories per serving: 115

Suitable for Vegetarians

Ingredients
- 12 sprigs dill, plus some chopped leaves, for topping
- 3 cups chicken broth, low-sodium
- 6 sprigs thyme
- 12 sprigs parsley
- 2 celery stalks, sliced thinly
- ½ white onion, diced
- 2 garlic cloves, minced
- 1 pound wild salmon fillet, skin removed and cut into 4 pieces
- 2 carrots, sliced thinly
- freshly ground pepper & salt to taste
- 1 wide strip lemon zest
- 1 pound potatoes, red-skinned, diced
- 2 bay leaves
- chopped chives, fresh, for topping
- ½ cup heavy cream

Directions

- Put the chicken broth in a microwave-safe bowl, preferably medium-sized &microwave for a couple of minutes, until very hot.
- In the meantime, scatter the carrots, potatoes, celery, garlic and onion in your slow cooker, preferably 6-quart or larger.
- Tie the parsley, dill, thyme, lemon zest and bay leaves together with twine & then add it to your slow cooker.
- Pour in the hot chicken broth; cover & cook for 3½ hours on high heat settings.
- Season the salmon with approximately ½ tsp. Pepper &1½ tsp. salt.
- Add the heavy cream into the vegetables; give everything a good stir, then submerge the salmon partially into the liquid.
- Cover &cook for half an hour more.
- Discard the herb bundle & season the chowder with pepper and salt.
- Top the chowder with dill and chives. Serve and enjoy.

Corned Beef and Cabbage

Prep Time: 15 minutes
Cook Time: 540 minutes
Total Time: 555 minutes
Servings: 8
Calories per serving: 472

Suitable for Vegetarians

Ingredients
- 1 corned beef brisket with spice packet (4 lbs.)
- 4 carrots, large, peeled &cut into matchstick pieces
- 6 oz. beer
- 1 onion, peeled &cut into pieces, preferably bite-sized
- 10 baby red potatoes, quartered
- 4 cups water
- ½ head cabbage, chopped coarsely

Directions

- Place the potatoes together with carrots & onion into the bottom of your slow cooker and then fill it with water; enough to cover everything and place the brisket over the vegetables.
- Transfer the beer on top of the brisket and then sprinkle the spices; cover & cook for 8 hours on high heat settings.
- During the last 60 minutes of your cooking, stir in the cabbage & cook for an hour more.

Paprika Goulash

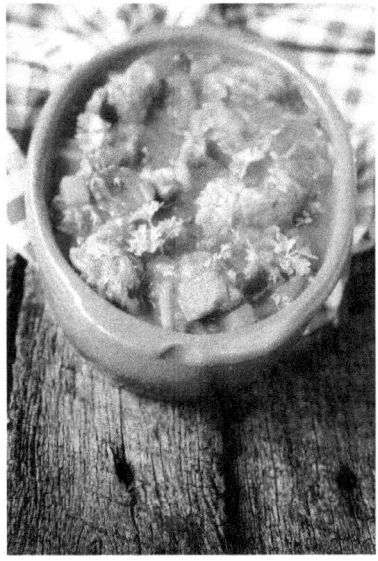

Prep Time: 15 minutes
Cook Time: 330 minutes
Total Time: 345 minutes
Servings: 8
Calories per serving: 149

Ingredients
- 4 tbsp. Hungarian paprika, smoked
- 3 sliced onions

- 1 tsp. black pepper, ground
- 2 tsp. thyme, dried
- 1 ¼ pounds pork loin, cubed
- 3 cloves garlic, chopped
- 1 tbsp. of olive oil
- ¾ cup tomato puree
- 1 cup yogurt, preferably Greek style
- ¾ cup water

Directions
- Combine the entire seasonings in a large-sized bowl.
- Coat the pork cubes in the seasoning mixture.
- Sauté garlic and onion in 1 tbsp. Oil for 4 minutes.
- Add in the pork and cook for 6 minutes.
- Transfer the pork and mixture to the slow cooker.
- In same pan, pour puree along with the water.
- Pour the puree mixture to the slow cooker.
- Cook on "low" for 8 hrs.
- Serve with yogurt.

Garlic Butter Tilapia

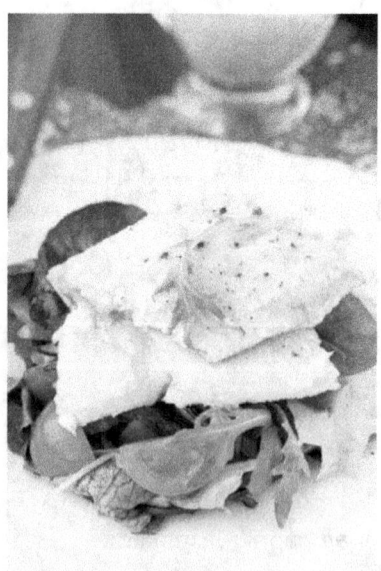

Prep Time: 5 minutes
Cook Time: 120 minutes
Total Time: 120 minutes
Servings: 3-4
Calories per serving: 116

Suitable for Vegetarians

Ingredients
- 4 tilapia fillets
- ground black pepper-and-salt, to taste
- 2 tbsp. garlic butter, sliced

Directions
- Arrange the tilapia fillets in large aluminium foil sheet and then season them with pepper and salt to taste; divide the butter pieces evenly over the fillets.
- Wrap the foil around the fish; sealing all sides completely & cook for 2 hours on high heat settings.
- Serve immediately.

Posole

Prep Time: 20 minutes
Cook Time: 395 minutes
Total Time: 415 minutes
Servings: 8
Calories per serving: 241

Ingredients
- 29 oz. Enchilada sauce
- 1 onion, sliced
- 2 lbs. rabbit, boneless, cut into 1" cubes
- ½ cup green chillies, diced
- 2 tsp. oregano, dried
- 31 oz. white hominy
- ½ tsp. cayenne pepper, or to taste
- 4 garlic cloves, minced
- ¼ cup cilantro, fresh, chopped
- 1 tbsp. canola oil

- ½ tsp. salt

Directions
- Over high heat settings in a large skillet; heat the canola oil.
- Add the rabbit; cook &stir for 5 minutes, until the meat is just browned on all sides.
- Place the meat in a slow cooker, preferably 4 quarts.
- Pour the enchilada sauce on top of the meat.
- Top with the garlic, chillies, onion, hominy, oregano and cayenne pepper.
- Pour in the water enough to fill your slow cooker.
- Cover & cook for 6 to 7 hours on high heat settings.
- Stir in the cilantro & salt; give everything a good stir.
- Cook for 30 more minutes on Low heat settings.

Barley and Chickpea Risotto

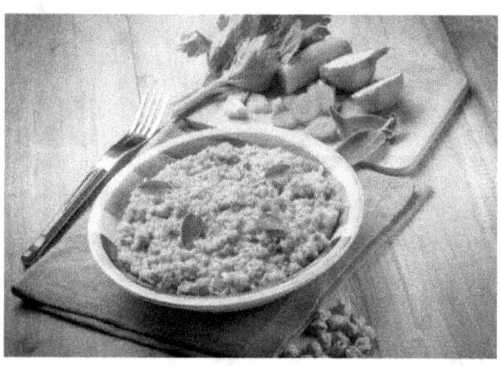

Prep Time: 10 minutes
Cook Time: 135 minutes
Total Time: 145 minutes
Servings: 4-6
Calories per serving: 237

Suitable for Vegetarians

Ingredients
- 15.5 ounces garbanzo beans, rinsed
- 1½ tbsp. extra virgin olive oil
- ½ head cauliflower, cut into small florets
- 1¼ cup pearl barley, rinsed
- ½ yellow onion, small, minced
- 4 sprigs thyme, fresh
- ⅓ cup Parmesan cheese, grated
- 3 cloves garlic, minced
- ¼ tsp. Ground black pepper
- 2 ½ cups vegetable or chicken broth, low-sodium
- 1¼ cups water
- 3 carrots, peeled &chopped
- 1½ tsp. Lemon juice, fresh
- ½ tsp. Salt

Directions
- Over moderate heat settings in a large saucepan; heat the oil.
- Add onion, carrots, cauliflower and garlic.
- Cook for 5 minutes, until the vegetables softens, stirring every now and then.
- Stir in the barley and thyme; cook for a couple of more minutes, stirring occasionally.
- Transfer the mixture to the bowl of your slow cooker.
- Stir in the garbanzo beans, water, broth, pepper and salt.
- Cook until most liquid is absorbed and barley is tender, for 2 to 2½ hours on high heat settings.
- Remove &discard the thyme sprigs and then stir in the lemon juice.
- Garnish with parsley and cheese. Serve and enjoy.

Supper

Rabbit Stew

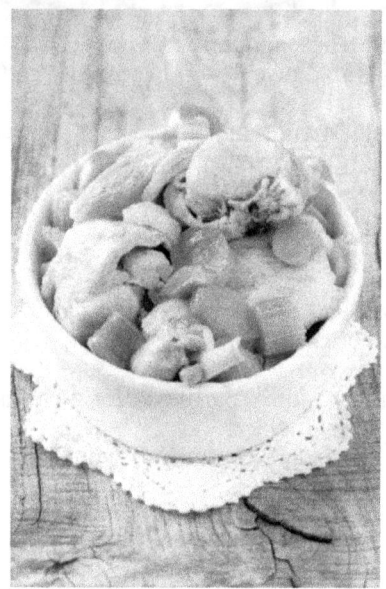

Prep Time: 15 minutes
Cook Time: 300 minutes
Total Time: 315 minutes
Servings: 10
Calories per serving: 381

Ingredients
- 4 carrots, medium, sliced
- 1 onion, chopped
- 3 celery stalks, chopped
- 1 tsp. thyme
- 4-5 lbs. rabbit, frozen
- 1 tbsp. basil
- 8-10 cups chicken broth

- 4 potatoes (skins on), medium, sliced
- ½ tsp. pepper
- 2 tsp. parsley
- 1 tsp. salt

Directions
- Add the vegetables and frozen rabbit to the bottom of your slow cooker.
- Pour broth over the ingredients completely.
- Add basil, thyme, pepper & salt.
- Cover & cook for 5 hours on high heat settings.
- Garnish with fresh parsley & serve hot.

Cheesy Mashed Potatoes

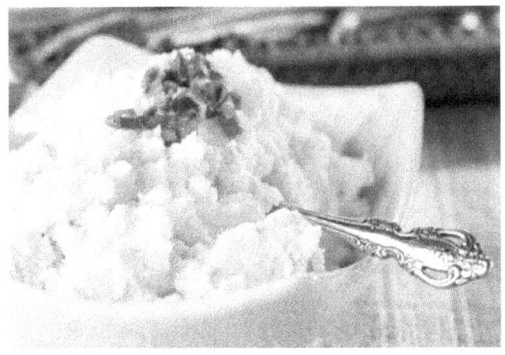

Prep Time: 5 minutes
Cook Time: 240 minutes
Total Time: 245 minutes
Servings: 8
Calories per serving: 255

Suitable for Vegetarians

Ingredients
- 1 cup Parmesan cheese, grated

- 3 - 4 lbs. potatoes, cleaned &cut into cubes
- 1 cup low sodium chicken broth
- 4 tbsp. unsalted butter
- ½ cup sour cream
- 1 cup whole milk
- 2 tbsp. chives, chopped for garnish
- 1 tsp. garlic powder
- pepper-and-salt, to taste

Directions
- Add the cubed potatoes into the bottom of your slow cooker.
- Add the milk, chicken broth, garlic powder, pepper and salt; give everything a good stir until evenly combined.
- Cover & cook until the potatoes are fork-tender, for 3½ to 4 hours on high heat settings.
- Add butter to the potatoes &mash them well using a potato masher.
- Stir in the Parmesan cheese and sour cream.
- Taste of pepper and salt and adjust the amount as required.
- Garnish with chives & serve hot.

Onion Dip in French Style

Prep Time: 10 minutes
Cook Time: 30 minutes
Total Time: 40 minutes
Servings: 4
Calories per serving: 151

Suitable for Vegetarians

Ingredients
- 1 clove garlic, minced
- ½ cup sour crème, low-fat
- 1 tbsp. Worcestershire sauce, low-sodium
- ½ white onion, chopped
- 1 tbsp. Olive oil
- ½ cup Greek yogurt, low-fat

- 1/16 tsp. of each kosher salt & black pepper

Directions
- Heat a small amount of oil in your slow cooker. Once hot; sauté the garlic and onion for a minute or two.
- Add in the rest of the ingredients.
- Cook for 30 minutes on low-heat settings.
- Garnish with chives (minced) and serve with vegetables.

Baked Beans

Prep Time: 10 minutes
Cook Time: 270 minutes
Total Time: 280 minutes
Servings: 4
Calories per serving: 254

Suitable for Vegetarians

Ingredients
- 4 oz. cooked ham, diced
- ½ cup barbeque sauce, hickory-flavoured
- 44 oz. great northern beans
- 1 tsp. dry mustard
- ½ cup brown sugar, packed
- 1 green bell pepper, diced
- ½ cup ketchup
- 1 onion, large, diced

Directions
- Mix the ketchup together with barbeque sauce, mustard &brown sugar in a slow cooker, preferably 4-quart or larger until smooth.
- Stir the green bell pepper, beans, ham & onion into the barbeque sauce mixture.
- Cook until thick, for 8 hours on low heat settings.
- Serve hot & enjoy.

Creamed Corn

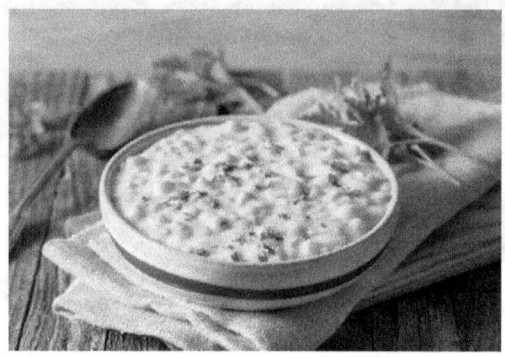

Prep Time: 10 minutes
Cook Time: 270 minutes
Total Time: 280 minutes
Servings: 4
Calories per serving: 192

Suitable for Vegetarians

Ingredients
- ½ cup butter
  - 1 package cream cheese (8 oz.)
  - 1¼ packages corn kernels, frozen (16 oz.)
  - 1 tbsp. white sugar
  - ½ cup milk
  - pepper and salt, to taste

Directions
- Combine corn together with butter, cream cheese, sugar & milk in a slow cooker.
- Season with pepper and salt, to taste.
- Cook for 4 hours on high heat settings.

Corn Chowder

Prep Time: 20 minutes
Cook Time: 510 minutes
Total Time: 530 minutes
Servings: 9
Calories per serving: 266

Ingredients
- 2 chicken bouillon cubes
- 5 potatoes, peeled & cubed
- 2 tbsp. butter
- 15.25 oz. whole kernel corn
- 2 onions, medium, chopped
- 3 celery stalks, chopped
- 2 cups ham, diced
- 12 oz. evaporated milk
- pepper & salt to taste

Directions
- Place ham together with the potatoes, corn, celery, onions, butter, pepper and salt taste in a slow cooker.
- Add water (enough to cover everything) and then add the chicken bouillon cubes.
- Cook for 8 to 9 hours on low-heat setting and then stir in the evaporated milk.
- Cook for half an hour more. Serve warm.

Split Pea Soup

Prep Time: 30 minutes
Cook Time: 360 minutes
Total Time: 390 minutes
Servings: 6
Calories per serving: 359

Ingredients

- ½ cup parsley, fresh, chopped, plus 8 to 10 parsley stems
- 2 carrots, chopped
- 1 pound green split peas, picked over &rinsed
- 2 celery stalks, chopped
- 1 leek, large, light green and white part only, halved lengthwise &sliced thinly crosswise
- ¼ cup plain yogurt, non-fat
- 1-1½ lbs. smoked turkey leg (1 whole)
- 4 sprigs thyme, fresh
- ½ cup peas, frozen, thawed
- freshly ground pepper & common salt, to taste

Optional Ingredients
- Crusty multigrain bread, for serving

Directions
- Tie the thyme together with parsley stems with kitchen string & then place it in a slow cooker.
- Add split peas together with carrots, leek, celery, ½ tsp. Pepper &1 tsp. Salt; give everything a good stir until evenly combined.
- Add the turkey leg followed by water (approximately 7 cups).
- Cover &cook for 6 to 8 hours on low heat settings, until the meat and split peas are tender.
- Discard the herb bundle; the bones and skin from the turkey leg; shredding the meat using two large forks.
- To make the soup smooth; strongly stir the soup and break up the peas. Feel free to add more water to make it thin, if desired.
- Stir in the freshly chopped parsley & approximately ¾ of the turkey meat, and season with pepper and salt.
- Ladle the soup into individual bowls.
- Add a small amount of water into the yogurt until thin and then spoon over the soup.
- Top with the leftover turkey and thawed peas.
- Serve warm with some bread.

Peach Cobbler

Prep Time: 15 minutes
Cook Time: 195 minutes
Total Time: 210 minutes
Servings: 4-6
Calories per serving: 316

Suitable for Vegetarians

Ingredients
- 6 oz. dark brown sugar
- ½ tsp. each freshly ground allspice, freshly grated nutmeg
- 3½ oz. rolled oats
- ½ tsp. baking powder
- 4 oz. all-purpose flour
- ¼ cup butter, unsalted, plus more for the cooker
- 20 oz. peach slices, frozen
- ¼ tsp. salt

Directions
- Combine flour together with oats, sugar, allspice, baking powder, nutmeg &salt in a bowl, preferably large-sized.
- Add butter; working into the dry ingredients until you get a crumbly texture.
- Fold in the frozen peach slices.
- Lightly butter the sides and bottom of your slow cooker.
- Add the mixture to the greased slow cooker &cook for 3 to 3½ hours on low heat settings.
- Serve immediately & enjoy.

Tapioca Pudding

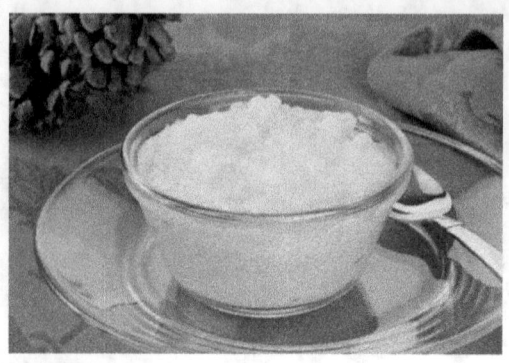

Prep Time: 15 minutes
Cook Time: 150 minutes
Total Time: 165 minutes
Servings: 8
Calories per serving: 190

Suitable for Vegetarians

Ingredients
- 4 cups whole milk
- ½ cup tapioca pearls, small
- 2 tsp. vanilla extract
- ⅔ cup white sugar
- 3 egg yolks, large
- ½ tsp. salt

Directions
- Whisk tapioca pearls together with milk, vanilla extract, sugar & salt in a slow cooker; whisk well until the sugar is completely dissolved.
- Close and cook for 2 hours on high-heat settings.
- In the meantime; whisk the egg yolks in a large bowl until smooth.
- Mix approximately 1 tbsp. Of the hot tapioca pudding into the egg yolks until combined thoroughly and continue to mix the hot tapioca pudding into the egg yolks until you get approximately 2 cups of the pudding and yolk mixture.
- Slowly transfer the yolk mixture in the slow cooker with the pudding until blended, whisk constantly for a couple of minutes, until you get a thick pudding like consistency.

- Place the lid on the cooker again and continue to cook for half an hour more, until you get your desired thickness of pudding.

Green Bean Risotto

Prep Time: 15 minutes
Cook Time: 150 minutes
Total Time: 165 minutes
Servings: 4
Calories per serving: 188

Suitable for Vegetarians

Ingredients
- 4 oz. green beans, frozen
- 1 oz. butter
- 2 garlic cloves, chopped
- 1 onion, chopped
- 8 oz. risotto rice
- 4 oz. frozen peas
- ground black pepper & salt to taste
- 2 tsp. pesto
- Basil leaves, for garnish
- 1.2 cups hot vegetable stock
- 1 tbsp. olive oil
- Parmesan shavings, for garnish

Directions
- Over moderate heat settings in a saucepan; heat the oil and butter. Once hot; fry the onion until the butter becomes soft & turns brownish, for a couple of minutes, stirring frequently.
- Stir in the rice and garlic; continue to cook for a minute more.
- Add approximately 150 ml. To the stock and then add pepper and salt to taste; bring everything together to a boil over moderate heat settings.
- Add to the pot of your slow cooker; cover & cook for 1¾ to 2 hours on low-heat settings.

- Stir in the leftover stock and pesto.
- Arrange the frozen green beans over the rice; close and cook for 20 to 30 more minutes.
- Garnish with Parmesan shavings &fresh basil leaves.

Serve warm and enjoy.

White Bean Stew

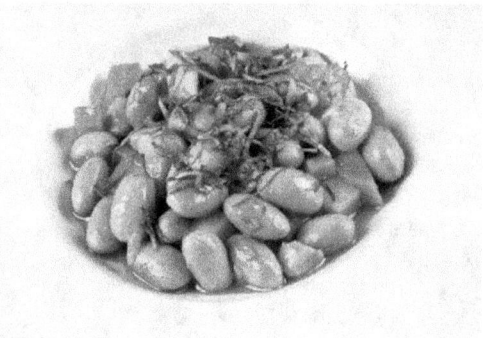

Prep Time: 20 minutes
Cook Time: 240 minutes
Total Time: 260 minutes
Servings: 10-12
Calories per serving: 291

Suitable for Vegetarians

Ingredients

- 5-6 cups of leafy greens (such as chard, spinach, kale) chopped roughly
- 2 lbs. great northern beans
- 1 tsp. each: oregano, thyme & dried rosemary
- 28 oz. tomatoes, diced
- 2 carrots, large, peeled &diced
- 1 onion, medium, diced
- 3 garlic cloves, chopped or minced
- 1 bay leaf

- 3 celery stalks, large & diced
- 10-12 cups water
- ground black pepper, to taste
- 2 tbsp. salt, or to taste

Directions
- Rinse the beans under cool running tap water.
- Add them with the garlic, diced carrots, onions, celery, bay leaf, dried rosemary, oregano and thyme to the bottom of your slow cooker and then add water (enough to cover everything).
- Cover & cook for 3 hours on high-heat settings.
- Carefully remove the lid and sprinkle pepper-and-salt to taste and then add the diced tomatoes.
- Let cook until beans are very soft, for 1 to 1½ more hours.
- Just before serving, don't forget to stir in the freshly chopped leafy greens.
- Serve the stew with some cooked rice, or polenta.

Cawl Cennin (Leek Soup)

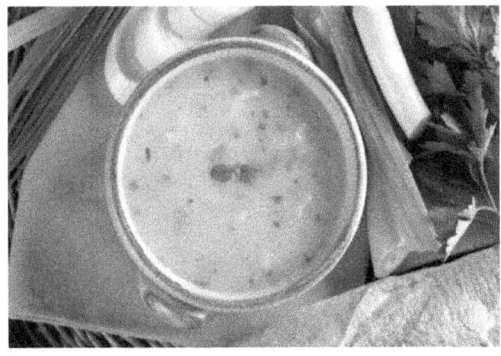

Prep Time: 20 minutes
Cook Time: 270 minutes
Total Time: 290 minutes
Servings: 4
Calories per serving: 248

Suitable for Vegetarians

Ingredients
- 4 leeks, large, sliced
- ¾ cup single cream
- 2½ cups vegetable stock
- 1 garlic clove, minced
- Parsley sprigs, fresh, for garnish
- 2 tbsp. Olive oil
- pepper & salt to taste

Directions
- Over moderate heat settings in a large frying pan; heat the oil. Once hot; carefully fry the garlic and leeks until begin to brown, for a couple of minutes.
- Transfer them to the bottom of your slow cooker and then add the stock. Finally sprinkle with pepper-and-salt to taste.
- Cook for 4½ hours on low-heat settings.
- Purée the soup in a blender until you get your desired consistency and then add the cream.
- Garnished the soup with fresh parsley & serve hot.

French Onion Soup

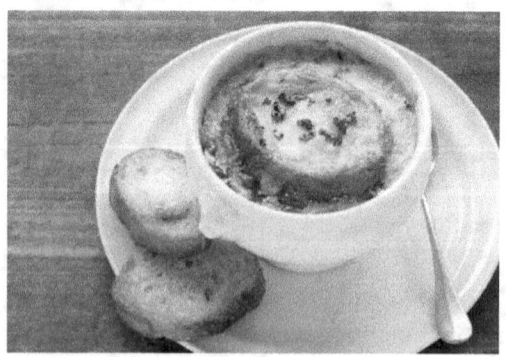

Prep Time: 30 minutes
Cook Time: 240 minutes
Total Time: 270 minutes
Servings: 4-6
Calories per serving: 335

Ingredients

- 8-12 slices Swiss cheese or gruyere
- 4 onions, yellow, skins removed & sliced thinly into rings
- 6 crusty French bread, slices
- 4 tbsp. butter
- 8 cups beef broth
- 2 tbsp. Garlic, minced
- 1 bay leaf

Directions

- Over medium-high heat settings in a large skillet or saucepan; heat the butter until completely melted. Once hot, sauté the onion rings until onions start to brown and are translucent, for 10 minutes.
- Cover & cook for a couple of more minutes and let them to caramelize a little more.
- Now, transfer the caramelized onions into the pot of your slow cooker.
- Add garlic, bay leaf and broth.
- Cover & cook for 4 hours on high-heat settings.
- During the last 30 minutes, preheat your oven to 435 F.
- Place the bread slices on a baking sheet in a single layer and then transfer it into the preheated oven. Bake for 4 to 5 minutes; flip and place the baking sheet again into the oven; bake until the bread is crunchy and dried, for 5 more minutes; set aside.
- Place the oven-safe bowls over the baking sheet; filling each of the bowls with soup.
- Place 2 Swiss cheese slices (slightly overlapping each other) over the soup.
- Bake until the cheese melts completely, for 8 to 10 minutes.
- Garnish with fresh parsley & serve with some crusty bread.

Seafood Cioppino

Prep Time: 20 minutes
Cook Time: 270 minutes
Total Time: 290 minutes
Servings: 8
Calories per serving: 205

Ingredients
- 1 pound haddock fillets, cut into 1" pieces
- 28 oz. Tomatoes, diced, undrained
- 1-2 tsp. Italian seasoning
- 3 celery ribs, chopped
- 2 onions, medium, chopped
- 6 oz. Tomato paste
- ½ cup vegetable broth
- 6 oz. Lump crabmeat
- 5 cloves garlic, minced
- 1 pound shrimp, uncooked, peeled & deveined
- 6 oz. Clams, chopped
- 1 bay leaf
- 2 tbsp. Parsley, fresh & minced
- 1 tbsp. Olive oil
- ½ tsp. Sugar

Directions
- Add & mix tomatoes together with tomato paste, celery ribs, onions, vegetable broth, olive oil, garlic clove, Italian seasoning, sugar and bay leaf in a slow cooker, preferably 4 quarts or larger.
- Cover &cook for 4 hours on low heat settings.
- Add the seafood; give everything a good stir.
- Cover &cook for 20 to 30 more minutes.
- Get rid of the bay leaf and then stir in the parsley. Serve warm and enjoy.

Broccoli and Cheese Soup

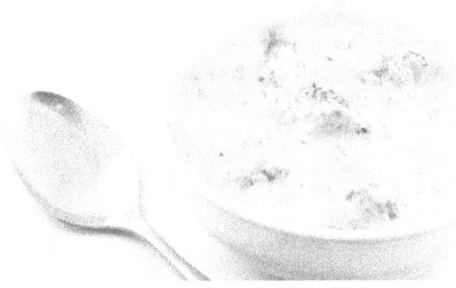

Prep Time: 15 minutes
Cook Time: 180 minutes
Total Time: 195 minutes
Servings: 6
Calories per serving: 190

Ingredients
- 6 tbsp. all-purpose flour
- ⅓ cup butter, sliced
- 24 oz. evaporated milk
- 2 garlic cloves, minced
- 5 cups chicken broth, low-sodium
- 1½ cups yellow onion, chopped
- 2 oz. Parmesan cheese, fresh, shredded finely
- 5 cups small broccoli florets, diced
- ½ cup heavy cream
- 12 oz. sharp cheddar cheese, freshly shredded
- Freshly ground black pepper & salt
- ⅛ tsp. dried thyme

Directions
- Over medium heat settings in a large skillet; heat the butter until completely melted and then sauté the onions until for a couple of minutes, begin to soften.
- Add garlic, all-purpose flour &lightly season with pepper and salt to taste; cook for a minute or two, stirring every now and then.

- While whisking, gradually pour in the evaporated milk; whisk well until completely smooth.
- Cook the mixture until it starts to thicken, stirring constantly and then pour the mixture along with diced broccoli, chicken broth & thyme into the slow cooker.
- Cover & cook for 2½ to 3 hours on high-heat settings.
- Turn off the heat settings & add the heavy cream; give everything a good stir and then add in the shredded Parmesan cheese and cheddar cheese; stir again.
- Season with pepper-and-salt to taste. Serve warm & enjoy.

Lentil Stew with Butternut Squash

Prep Time: 5 minutes
Cook Time: 480 minutes
Total Time: 485 minutes
Servings: 8
Calories per serving: 191

Suitable for Vegetarians

Ingredients
- 1 bag brown lentils
- 3 stalks celery, large
- 1 butternut squash, large
- ¼ tsp. ground black pepper
- 1 can vegetable broth
- ½ tsp. rosemary, dried
- 1 onion, large
- ¼ cups parsley leaves, fresh, loosely packed, for garnish
- 4 cups water
- 1 oz. parmesan cheese, for garnish
- ¾ tsp. salt

Directions
- Combine onion together with squash, celery, rosemary, lentils, broth, water, ¼ tsp. Freshly ground black pepper and ¾ tsp. Salt in the bowl of your slow cooker.

- Cover & cook for 8 hours on low-heat settings.
- Spoon the lentil stew into individual serving bowls and then garnish each bowl with Parmesan shavings, lastly sprinkle chopped parsley over the top. Serve warm and enjoy.

Butternut Squash Stew

Prep Time: 10 minutes
Cook Time: 420 minutes
Total Time: 430 minutes
Servings: 4
Calories per serving: 255

Suitable for Vegetarians

Ingredients
- 1 can whole tomatoes
- 2 tsp. ground cumin
- ½ butternut squash, medium
- 1½ tsp. ground ginger
- ¼ tsp. ground cinnamon
- 1 cup couscous
- ½ cup raisins
- 1 red onion
- ¼ cup cilantro, fresh
- pepper and salt, to taste

Directions
- Place tomatoes together with the juices in a slow cooker, preferably 5 to 6-quart or larger and slightly break them up.
- Add raisins together with ginger, cumin, cinnamon, ¼ tsp. Pepper & ½ tsp. Salt or the taste; mix until evenly combined.
- Add the squash and onion; give everything a good stir; cover &cook until the squash is tender, for 6 to 7 hours on low heat settings.
- Prepare the couscous at least 10 minutes before serving and then fold in the cilantro.
- Serve the squash stew over couscous and enjoy.

Red Lentil Curry

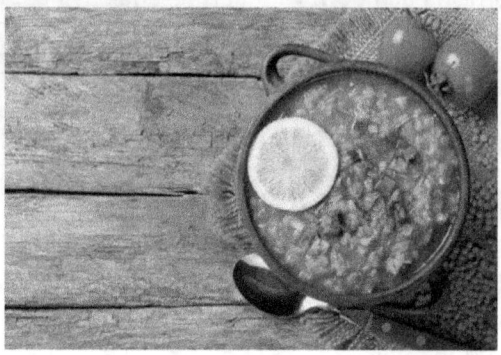

Prep Time: 5 minutes
Cook Time: 270 minutes
Total Time: 275 minutes
Servings: 16
Calories per serving: 255

Suitable for Vegetarians

Ingredients
- 4 cups brown lentils; rinsed
- 58 oz. tomato puree
- 1 tbsp. garam masala
- 2 onions, diced
- 1 tbsp. ginger, minced
- 5 tbsp. red curry paste
- 1½ tsp. turmeric
- 4 garlic cloves, minced
- cilantro, fresh for garnishing
- ½ cup coconut cream or milk
- 4 tbsp. butter, unsalted
- 2 cups water
- rice, for serving
- 2 tsp. sugar
- 1 tsp. salt or to taste

Directions
- Place the rinsed lentils in a Crockpot, preferably large size.

- Add the ginger, garlic, diced onions, curry paste, butter, garam masala, turmeric, cayenne &sugar; give everything a good stir until evenly combined.
- Add tomato puree on top of the lentils.
- Add water; stir well and ensure the lentils are completely covered with the liquid.
- Cover &cook for 4 to 5 hours on high-heat settings.
- Don't forget to check it occasionally during the cooking time and if the lentils are soaking up the liquid completely, feel free to add more of tomato puree or water.
- Pour the coconut milk; stir well and then just before serving, sprinkle with freshly chopped cilantro.
- Serve with naan bread or over rice.

Vindaloo Vegetables

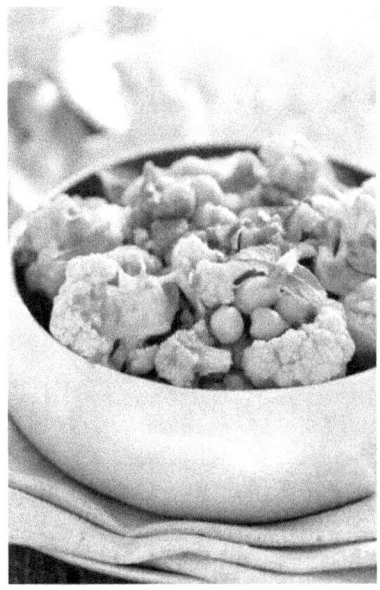

Prep Time: 15 minutes
Cook Time: 35 minutes
Total Time: 50 minutes
Servings: 6

Calories per serving: 159

Suitable for Vegetarians
Ingredients
- 4 cups cauliflower florets, small
- 1 tbsp. ginger, peeled & chopped
- 3 garlic cloves, peeled
- 1 date, pitted, chopped coarsely
- ½ tsp. cayenne pepper or to taste
- 1½ tsp. ground coriander
- ½ tsp. turmeric
- 1¼ tsp. ground cumin
- ¼ tsp. cardamom
- 1 yellow onion, large, chopped
- 2 carrots, small & sliced thinly
- 1 bell pepper, small, seeded & diced
- 6 oz. tomato paste
- 1 cup green peas, frozen, thawed
- freshly ground black pepper and salt, to taste

Directions
- Combine garlic together with coriander, ginger, date & ½ cup water in a food processor or blender; process on high settings until smooth, set aside.
- Over moderate heat settings in a wok or large non-stick pot; add carrots and onions with 1 tbsp. Water; cover & cook for a couple of minutes, until softened. To prevent burning, feel free to add more of water and don't forget to stir occasionally.
- Add the prepared spice paste; cook & stir for a couple of minutes, then add in the cauliflower.
- Cover & decrease the heat settings to low.
- Put the tomato paste & 1¼ cups of water in the same food processor or blender; blend until completely mixed.
- Add the tomato paste mixture to the vegetables; cover & cook for a couple of minutes.
- Add in the bell pepper and season with salt and pepper; continue to cook for a couple of minutes, until the vegetables are tender, covered.
- Add the peas & let heat for a few minutes.
- Serve as it is or over some steamed cooked rice.

Mexican Quinoa

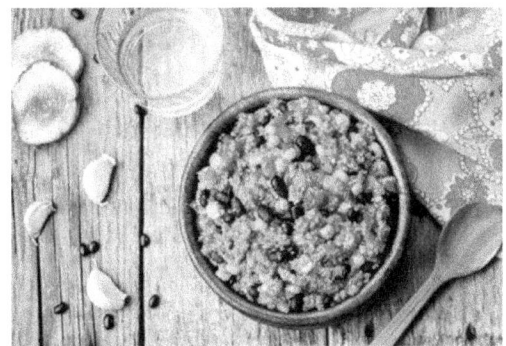

Prep Time: 10 minutes
Cook Time: 240 minutes
Total Time: 250 minutes
Servings: 6-8
Calories per serving: 298

Suitable for Vegetarians

Ingredients
- 1 tsp. garlic, minced
- 1½ lbs. butternut squash, peeled & de-seeded
- 1 cup corn, frozen
- 14.5 oz. petite diced tomatoes, fire-roasted
- 1 jalapeno, small
- 15.25 oz. black beans, rinsed
- 1 cup quinoa, uncooked, rinsed
- 38 oz. each mild red enchilada sauce
- 1 cup chicken or vegetable broth
- 1.25 oz. taco seasoning

Optional Ingredients
- Fresh lime juice, shredded cheddar cheese, chopped cilantro and/or sour cream for topping

Directions
- Cut the butternut squash into small cubes & then place them in a slow cooker.

- Add the fire-roasted petite diced tomatoes, rinsed black beans, diced jalapeno, corn, enchilada sauce, minced garlic, chicken or vegetable broth & taco seasoning; give everything a good stir.
- Cover & cook until the butternut squash is tender and the quinoa is cooked through, for 3 to 4 hours on high-heat settings.
- Uncover, stir well & set aside for half an hour until the quinoa absorbs most of the liquid.
- Season with any extra spices and/or pepper and salt, if desired.
- Top the bowls with toppings such as fresh lime juice, shredded cheese, sour cream & cilantro.

Lemon Rosemary Lentil Soup

Prep Time: 15 minutes
Cook Time: 360 minutes
Total Time: 375 minutes
Servings: 6-8
Calories per serving: 298

Ingredients
- 6 carrots, diced
- ⅛ tsp. cayenne pepper
- 3 cups red lentils
- 1 onion, large, diced
- 4 cups chicken broth
- 1 yellow pepper, chopped
- 4 garlic cloves, minced
- juice and zest of 1 lemon, fresh
- 2¾ cups water
- 1 tbsp. rosemary, fresh, chopped
- 1½ tsp. salt

Directions
- Add the entire ingredients (except the rosemary and lemon juice and zest) in a slow cooker.
- Cook for 6 hours on low-heat settings.

- Once the cooking cycle completes; stir in the lemon juice, zest &rosemary.
- Season with more of pepper and salt, to taste.
- Ladle the soup into individual bowls & garnish with extra chopped rosemary. Serve hot and enjoy.

Black Bean Soup

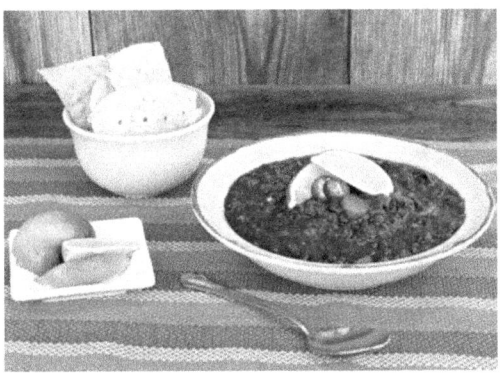

Prep Time: 10 minutes
Cook Time: 240 minutes
Total Time: 250 minutes
Servings: 6-8
Calories per serving: 250

Suitable for Vegetarians

Ingredients
- 2 red bell peppers, cored & chopped
- 1 yellow or white onion, large, chopped
- 2 tsp. chilli powder
- 1-2 jalapeno peppers, seeded & diced
- 2 carrots, chopped
- 4 cups vegetable stock, best quality
- 2 tsp. ground cumin
- 60 oz. black beans, rinsed
- 1 bay leaf
- 5 garlic cloves, minced

- ½ tsp. cayenne pepper
- 2 tsp. salt

Directions
- Combine the entire ingredients together in a slow cooker bowl; give everything a good stir.
- Cover &cook until the entire vegetables are tender and cooked through, for 3 to 4 hours on high-heat settings.
- Get rid of the bay leaf.
- Ladle the soup into individual bowls and serve hot.

Butter Chickpeas and Tofu

Prep Time: 15 minutes
Cook Time: 240 minutes
Total Time: 255 minutes
Servings: 4-6
Calories per serving: 328

Suitable for Vegetarians

Ingredients
- 1 package firm tofu (12 oz.); rinsed
- 4 cloves garlic, minced
- 1 tbsp. garam masala
- 2 cups coconut milk
- 1 onion, medium, diced
- 15 oz. garbanzo beans, rinsed
- 1 tsp. chilli powder
- ½ tsp. ground ginger
- 1 tbsp. curry powder
- ⅛ cup cilantro, chopped finely
- 1 cup tomato puree
- pepper & salt, to taste
- 1 tsp. Olive oil

Directions
- Wrap the rinsed tofu in a paper towel &place it on a clean cutting board.

- Put something heavy over the tofu; set aside for a couple of minutes until the water is drained out.
- Over medium-high heat settings in a saucepan; heat the olive oil and then sauté the onion for a couple of minutes, until soft & translucent.
- Add the garlic; give everything a good stir until evenly combined.
- Whisk in the ground ginger, coconut milk, curry powder, garam masala, chilli powder, tomato puree &a pinch of pepper and salt.
- Cook for a couple of minutes, until slightly thick.
- In the meantime, finely cube the drained tofu.
- Place the garbanzo beans and tofu in a slow cooker.
- Pour the prepared sauce over the top.
- Cook until thick, for 4 to 5 hours on low heat settings. Just before serving, don't forget to stir in the cilantro.
- Serve with naan and/or some steamed cooked rice.

Chana Masala

Prep Time: 5 minutes
Cook Time: 540 minutes
Total Time: 545 minutes
Servings: 6
Calories per serving: 170

Suitable for Vegetarians

Ingredients

- 30 oz. chickpeas
- 1 tsp. ground coriander
- 28 oz. tomatoes, diced
- 1 onion, large, diced
- 6 oz. tomato paste
- ½ tsp. cayenne pepper or to taste
- 2 tsp. garam masala
- 1 tsp. turmeric
- 2 tsp. garlic powder
- ⅓ cup cilantro leaves, fresh, chopped

- 1 tsp. cumin
- 4 cups water
- basmati rice, cooked, for serving
- 1 tsp. sea salt

Directions
- Combine the entire ingredients (except the chickpeas) in a slow cooker; give everything a good stir; cover and cook for 6 to 8 hours on low-heat settings.
- Once done, add in the chickpeas & cook until tender, for 2 more hours.
- Serve over some prepared basmati rice.

Chicken Chilli

Prep Time: 5 minutes
Cook Time: 480 minutes
Total Time: 485 minutes
Servings: 10
Calories per serving: 266

Ingredients
- 15.5 ounce Kidney beans, rinsed
- ½ cup sweet onion, diced
- 2 cloves garlic, minced
- 1.5 lbs chicken breast fillets (approximately 2 -3), cut into pieces, preferably bite-sized
- ½ tsp. Cayenne pepper or to taste
- 14.5 ounce fire roasted tomatoes
- ½ tsp. Black pepper
- 2 tbsp. Chilli powder
- ½ tsp. Cumin
- 6 Oz tomato paste
- ¼ cup cheddar cheese, reduced fat, for garnish
- 1½ cups vegetable broth or chicken broth, low sodium, fat free
- Sea salt, to taste

Directions

- Combine the entire ingredients into the bottom of your slow cooker.
- Cover & cook for 8 hours on low-heat settings.
- Spoon the chilli into individual bowls & garnish with a small amount of cheddar cheese &diced onion. Serve hot & enjoy.

Chicken Fajitas

Prep Time: 5 minutes
Cook Time: 240 minutes
Total Time: 245 minutes
Servings: 6
Calories per serving: 364

Rub Ingredients
- 1 tsp. chilli powder
- ½ tsp. garlic powder
- 1 tsp. hot smoked paprika
- ½ tsp. white or black pepper
- 1 tsp. red chilli flakes, dried
- ½ tsp. cayenne pepper
- 1 tsp. onion powder
- ½ tsp. salt
- 1 tsp. dried oregano

Fajita Ingredients
- 1 yellow & orange bell pepper, preferably sliced into 1" pieces
- 2 large chicken breasts, boneless
- 1 red bell pepper, sliced into 1-inch pieces
- 14.5 oz. organic tomatoes with green chillies
- 1 large white onion, sliced into ½" pieces
- 6 whole wheat tortillas
- 1 tbsp. Olive oil, divided

Directions
- Combine the entire rub ingredients together in a large-sized pie plate.

- Now, rub both sides of the chicken breasts with 2 tsp. Olive oil and then dredges both sides of the chicken breasts with blackening spice; discarding any excess rub.
- Layer ½ of tomatoes, onions and peppers in a slow cooker.
- Top with the chicken pieces, leftover tomatoes, onions and peppers.
- Cover & cook for 3 to 4 hours on high-heat settings.
- Serve on tortillas along with avocado, cilantro & lime wedges.

Super food Soup

Prep Time: 5 minutes
Cook Time: 420 minutes
Total Time: 425 minutes
Servings: 8
Calories per serving: 157

Ingredients
- 30 oz. black beans, rinsed
- 1 sweet potato, large, cut into ½" cubes
- 2 cups carrots, sliced
- 1 garlic clove, minced
- ½ cup cilantro, fresh, chopped
- 1 cup green beans, fresh or frozen
- ½ tsp. red pepper flakes, crushed
- 1 tsp. chilli powder
- 2 cups vegetable juice
- 1 tsp. cumin
- 2 cups vegetable broth, low-sodium
- 1 onion, small, diced
- ½ tsp. black pepper
- salt to taste

Directions
- Place everything together in the bottom of your slow cooker; give everything a good stir until evenly combined.
- Cover & cook until the veggies are tender, for 6 to 8 hours on low-heat settings.

- Serve warm & enjoy.

Pinto & Black Bean Chilli

Prep Time: 15 minutes
Cook Time: 270 minutes
Total Time: 285 minutes
Servings: 8
Calories per serving: 217.3
Suitable for Vegetarians

Ingredients
- 29 Oz diced tomatoes
- 1 pound of turkey (ground); cut into pieces
- 14.5 Oz black beans
- 1 chopped green pepper
- 14.5 Oz rinsed pinto beans, rinsed
- 1 tsp. oregano
- ½ tsp. cumin
- 1 clove garlic, minced
- 1 ½ tsp. cayenne pepper
- 1 tsp. of black pepper
- 1 onion, medium, chopped

Directions
- Put everything together in the bottom of your slow cooker; give everything a good stir until mixed well.
- Add water; cover & cook for 4 hours on High-heat settings.
- Serve warm & enjoy.

Quinoa Risotto

Prep Time: 5minutes
Cook Time: 240minutes

Total Time: 245minutes
Servings: 6
Calories per serving: 217

Ingredients
- 2 cups peas, frozen
- 1½ lbs. asparagus, trimmed & quartered
- 2 cups quinoa, rinsed
- 4 cups chicken broth, low-sodium
- 2 garlic cloves, minced
- 1½ lbs. chicken breasts, boneless, skinless
- 3 carrots, large, sliced into rounds
- freshly ground black pepper & salt, to taste

Directions
- Combine chicken together with quinoa, carrots, chicken broth and garlic in the cooking pot of your slow-cooker.
- Season with pepper and salt to taste.
- Cover & cook until the chicken is cooked through, for 4 hours on high-heat settings; shred the chicken using two forks and then add peas and asparagus to the slow cooker; cook until tender, for half an hour more.
- Pour on top of the leftover chicken broth; give everything a good stir until creamy.
- Serve warm & enjoy.

Chicken Soup

Prep Time: 5 minutes
Cook Time: 420 minutes
Total Time: 425 minutes
Servings: 8
Calories per serving: 346

Ingredients
- 3 tsp. dried thyme
- 2 pounds uncooked chicken thighs or breasts, skinless, boneless; cut into 2" pieces
- 1 tsp. dried oregano
- 4 carrots, sliced

- 1 onion, small, diced
- 2 garlic cloves, minced
- 1-2 tbsp. lemon juice, freshly squeezed to taste
- ½ tsp. red pepper flakes, crushed or to taste
- 1 cup celery, sliced
- 6 cups fat-free chicken broth, low-sodium
- ¼ cup Italian parsley, fresh, chopped, to serve
- 1 bay leaf
- ½ tsp. black pepper
- 1 tsp. sea salt

Directions
- Add garlic together with vegetables to the bottom of your slow cooker; add chicken over the top and then sprinkle with oregano, thyme, chilli flakes, pepper and salt.
- Pour in the stock and then add the bay leaf.
- Cover & cook until the carrots are tender, on low-heat settings for 6 to 8 hours.
- During the last 15 minutes of your cooking; stir in 1tbsp. Of the lemon juice.
- Taste & feel free to add more of lemon juice, if desired.
- Serve& enjoy.

Spinach and Artichoke Chicken

Prep Time: 5 minutes
Cook Time: 420 minutes
Total Time: 425 minutes
Servings: 4
Calories per serving: 246

Ingredients
- 4 bone-in with skin whole chicken breasts (6-8 oz.)
- 8 cups spinach, loosely packed, chopped
- 1 cup chicken broth
- 4 tbsp. cream cheese, reduced-fat but not fat free
- ¼ sweet onion, finely chopped
- 3 garlic cloves, fresh, chopped
- 6- 8 artichoke hearts, chopped
- 1 cup cherry tomatoes or chopped grapes

- 4 tbsp. parmesan cheese, shredded
- pepper and salt, to taste

Directions
- Place spinach together with chicken breasts and chicken broth into the cooking bowl of your slow cooker.
- Sprinkle with onion, garlic, pepper and salt.
- Cover &cook for 6 to 8 hours on low-heat settings.
- Just before serving, remove the cooked chicken breasts gently from the slow cooker &place them on individual serving plates.
- Stir in the artichokes, Parmesan cheese and cream cheese; stir until completely creamy.
- Spoon the sauce on top of the chicken.
- Top with tomatoes and then sprinkle with more of Parmesan cheese, if desired.

Fiesta Chicken Soup

Prep Time: 5 minutes
Cook Time: 420 minutes
Total Time: 425 minutes
Servings: 10
Calories per serving: 192

Ingredients
- 2 chicken breast fillets, skinless, cut into cubes
- 1 tbsp. chilli powder
- 14.5 oz. diced tomatoes
- ½ cup onion, diced
- 1 clove garlic, minced
- 2½ cups fat-free chicken broth, low sodium
- 1 cup corn, fresh or frozen
- ½ cup cilantro, freshly chopped
- juice from 1 lime, fresh
- 4.5 oz. green chilli peppers, diced
- 1 tsp. cumin
- ½ tsp. black pepper
- sea salt, to taste

Directions
- Put everything together to the bottom of your slow cooker; give everything a good stir until evenly combined.
- Cover & cook 6 to 8 hours on low-heat settings.
- Serve hot & enjoy.

Curly Coley

Prep Time: 10 minutes
Cook Time: 120 minutes
Total Time: 130 minutes
Servings: 4-6
Calories per serving: 100

Suitable for Vegetarians

Ingredients
- 14.5 oz. tomatoes, chopped
- 1 onion, coarsely chopped
- 3 garlic cloves, chopped
- 2 coley fillets
- 6 mushrooms, sliced
- Parsley to taste
- 1 tbsp. olive oil

Directions
- Preheat your slow cooker over high-heat setting in advance.
- Once hot; add olive oil and cook the onions & garlic for a couple of minutes.
- Add the chopped tomatoes; fill it with water to the slow cooker.
- Garnish with parsley.
- Finally, add the sliced mushroom and Coley; give everything a good stir until evenly mixed.
- Cook for 2 hours on high-heat settings.
- Serve the cooked Coley with some pasta or rice or alone in a warm bowl.

Butternut Squash and Parsnip Soup

Prep Time: 5 minutes
Cook Time: 360 minutes
Total Time: 365 minutes
Servings: 4-6
Calories per serving: 132

Ingredients
- 2 cups parsnip, chopped
- 3 packages butternut squash, frozen, thawed (12 oz.)
- 2 cups sweet onions, chopped
- 1½ cups granny smith apple, peeled & chopped
- 2 cups fat-free chicken broth, lower-sodium
- ⅛ tsp. paprika
- 2 tbsp. whipping cream
- ⅛ tsp. ground cumin
- 3 cups water
- 1 tsp. freshly ground black pepper
- ¼ tsp. salt

Optional Ingredients
- 8 tsp. chives, fresh, chopped
- ½ cup light sour cream

Directions
- Combine onion together with apple, parsnip, butternut squash, black pepper, salt, chicken broth & water in a slow cooker.
- Cover & cook for 6 hours on low-heat settings.
- Place 1/4thof the squash mixture in a blender.
- Remove the middle piece of blender lid and then secure the lid on the blender.
- Place a clean towel over opening in blender lid.
- Blend on high settings until smooth.
- Pour the mixture into a large-sized bowl.
- Repeat the procedure with leftover squash mixture. Stir in the paprika, whipping cream & cumin.
- Ladle the soup into individual bowls& then tops each serving with chives and sour cream, if desired.

Lemon Rosemary Beets

Prep Time: 5 minutes
Cook Time: 480 minutes
Total Time: 485 minutes
Servings: 5-6
Calories per serving: 112

Ingredients
- 5-6 beets, peeled &cut into wedges
- 2 rosemary sprigs
- 1 tbsp. cider vinegar
- 2 tbsp. fresh lemon juice
- ½ tsp. grated lemon rind
- 2 tbsp. extra-virgin olive oil
- ½ tsp. freshly ground black pepper
- 2 tbsp. honey
- ¾ tsp. salt

Directions
- Place everything together (except the lemon rind) into the cooking pot of your slow cooker.
- Cover & cook until the beets are tender, for 8 hours on low-heat settings.
- Remove & discard the rosemary sprigs; add the lemon rind, give everything a good stir.
- Serve hot & enjoy.

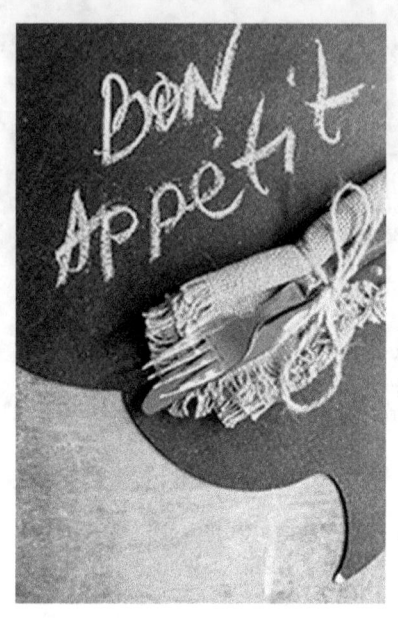

100 Slow Cooker Recipes for you: Cookbook how to Cook healthy meals for Weight Loss

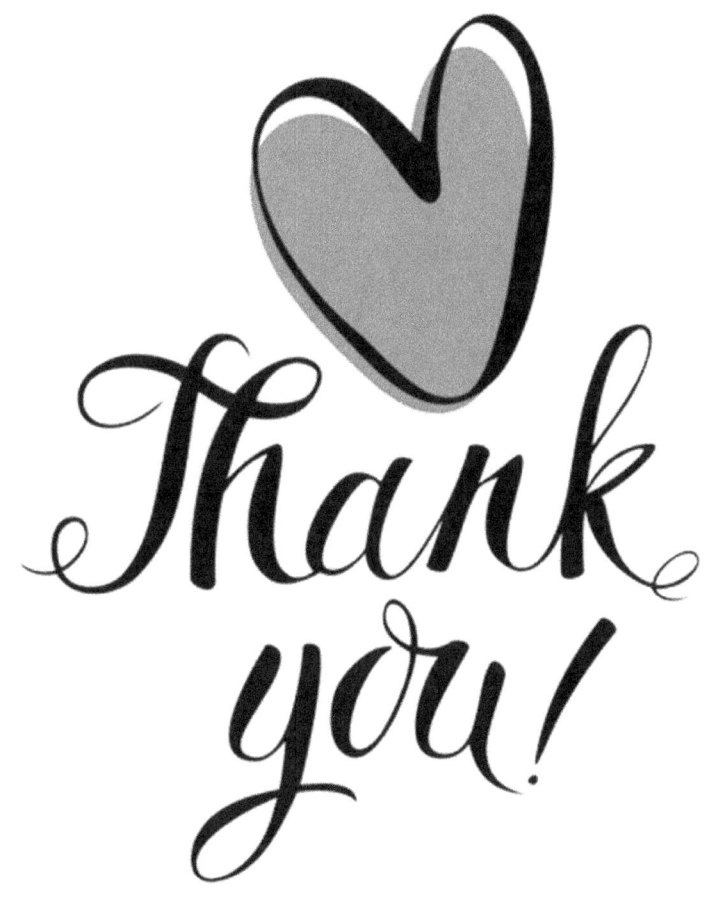

Helena Smith

www.helsmts@gmail.com

**Copyright 2018 by Helena Smith –
All rights reserved.**

All rights Reserved. No part of this publication or the information in it may be quoted from, or reproduced in any form by means such as printing, scanning, photocopying or otherwise without prior written permission of the copyright holder.

Disclaimer and Terms of Use: Effort has been made to ensure that the information in this book is accurate and complete, however, the author and the publisher do not warrant the accuracy of the information, text and graphics contained within the book due to the rapidly changing nature of science, research, known and unknown facts and internet. The Author and the publisher do not hold any responsibility for errors, omissions or contrary interpretation of the subject matter herein. This book is presented solely for motivational and informational purposes only.

www.ingramcontent.com/pod-product-compliance
Lightning Source LLC
Chambersburg PA
CBHW052326220526
45472CB00001B/293